Time Use Studies and Unpaid Care Work

Routledge/UNRISD Research in Gender and Development

1. New Perspectives on Gender and Migration
Livelihood, Rights and Entitlements
Edited by Nicola Piper

2. Gendered Peace
Women's Struggles for Post-War Justice and Reconciliation
Edited by Donna Pankhurst

3. Global Perspectives on Gender Equality
Reversing the Gaze
Edited by Naila Kabeer and Agneta Stark with Edda Magnus

4. Social Justice and Gender Equality
Rethinking Development Strategies and Macroeconomic Policies
Edited by Günseli Berik, Yana van der Meulen Rodgers, and Ann Zammit

5. Governing Women
Women's Political Effectiveness in Contexts of Democratization and Governance Reform
Edited by Anne Marie Goetz

6. The Gendered Impacts of Liberalization
Towards "Embedded Liberalism"?
Edited by Shahra Razavi

7. Time Use Studies and Unpaid Care Work
Edited by Debbie Budlender

United Nations Research Institute for Social Development

UNRISD is an autonomous agency engaging in multidisciplinary research on the social dimensions of contemporary problems affecting development. Its work is guided by the conviction that, for effective development policies to be formulated, an understanding of the social and political context is crucial. The Institute attempts to provide governments, development agencies, grass-roots organizations and scholars with a better understanding of how development policies and processes of economic, social and environmental change affect different social groups. Working through an extensive network of national research centres, UNRISD aims to promote original research and strengthen research capacity in developing countries.

Current research programmes include: Civil Society and Social Movements; Democracy, Governance and Well-Being; Gender and Development; Identities, Conflict and Cohesion; Markets, Business and Regulation; and Social Policy and Development. For further information on UNRISD work, visit www.unrisd.org.

Time Use Studies and Unpaid Care Work

Edited by Debbie Budlender

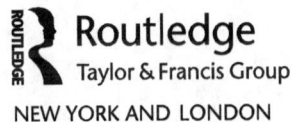

NEW YORK AND LONDON

First published 2010
by Routledge
605 Third Avenue, New York, NY 10017

Simultaneously published in the UK
by Routledge
4 Park Square, Milton Park, Abingdon, Oxon OX14 4RN

Routledge is an imprint of the Taylor & Francis Group, an informa business

First published in paperback 2012

© 2010 United Nations Research Institute for Social Development (UNRISD)

The right of Debbie Budlender to be identified as the author of the editorial material, and of the authors for their individual chapters, has been asserted by them in accordance with sections 77 and 78 of the Copyright, Designs and Patents Act 1988.

Typeset in Sabon by IBT Global.

All rights reserved. No part of this book may be reprinted or reproduced or utilised in any form or by any electronic, mechanical, or other means, now known or hereafter invented, including photocopying and recording, or in any information storage or retrieval system, without permission in writing from the publishers.

Trademark Notice: Product or corporate names may be trademarks or registered trademarks, and are used only for identification and explanation without intent to infringe.

Library of Congress Cataloging-in-Publication Data
 Time use studies and unpaid care work / edited by Debbie Budlender.
   p. cm. — (Routledge/UNRISD research in gender and development ; 7)
 Includes bibliographical references and index.
 1. Time management—Cross-cultural studies. 2. Caregivers—Cross-cultural studies. 3. Caregivers—Salaries, etc.—Cross-cultural studies. I. Budlender, Debbie.
   HD69.T54T488 2010
   362'.0425068—dc22
   2010005910

ISBN13: 978-0-415-88224-8 (hbk)
ISBN13: 978-0-203-84614-8 (ebk)
ISBN13: 978-0-415-81102-6 (pbk)

Contents

List of Figures	vii
List of Tables	xi
List of Acronyms and Abbreviations	xix
Foreword	xxi

1   What do Time Use Studies Tell Us about Unpaid Care Work? Evidence from Seven Countries   1
DEBBIE BUDLENDER

2   Tanzania: Care in the Context of HIV and AIDS   46
DEBBIE BUDLENDER

3   South Africa: When Marriage and the Nuclear Family Are Not the Norm   69
DEBBIE BUDLENDER

4   Unpaid Care Work: Analysis of the Indian Time Use Data   92
NEETHA N. AND RAJNI PALRIWALA

5   Republic of Korea: Analysis of Time Use Survey on Work and Care   118
MI-YOUNG AN

6   Analysis of Time Use Surveys on Work and Care in Japan   142
YUKO TAMIYA AND MASATO SHIKATA

7   The Case of Nicaragua   171
ISOLDA ESPINOSA GONZÁLEZ

8	Unpaid Care Work in the City of Buenos Aires VALERIA ESQUIVEL	197
Index		223

Figures

1.1	Participation rates by SNA category, country and sex.	13
1.2	Mean time spent per day on activities by SNA category, country and sex for full sample population.	15
1.3	Mean time spent per day on activities by SNA category, country and sex for actors.	17
1.4	Composition of hours spent on SNA and unpaid care work by sex.	19
1.5	Participation rates by sub-category of unpaid care work, country and sex.	21
1.6	Mean time spent per day on activities by sub-category of unpaid care work, country and sex for full sample population.	22
1.7	Mean time spent per day on sub-categories of unpaid care work by country and sex for actors.	23
1.8	Care dependency ratios.	33
1.9	Components of care dependency ratios.	34
1.10	Value of unpaid care work and care of persons as a percentage of GDP.	39
1.11	Value of unpaid care work as a percentage of paid work in the economy.	41
1.12	Value of unpaid care work as percentage of personal tax.	42
2.1	Time spent on paid and unpaid work by sex.	51
2.2	Percentage of people doing person care and paid work by sex.	58

viii *Figures*

2.3	Distribution of time spent on unpaid care work by sex.	64
2.4	Distribution of time spent on person care.	64
3.1	Time spent on paid and unpaid work by sex.	74
3.2	Percentage of people doing person care and paid work by sex.	81
3.3	Distribution of time spent on unpaid care work by sex.	86
3.4	Distribution of time spent on person care.	87
4.1	Mean hours per day spent by actors on SNA and extended SNA by sex and location.	96
4.2	Mean hours spent daily on SNA and extended SNA by marital status.	98
4.3	Distribution of number of persons across various time slots spent on unpaid care work.	104
4.4	Distribution of population by sex and time spent on person care.	112
5.1	Time spent on activities by sex in 1999 and 2004.	122
5.2	Distribution of time spent on unpaid care work by sex, 1999.	134
5.3	Distribution of time spent on person care by sex, 1999.	134
5.4	Distribution of time spent on unpaid care work by sex, 2004.	135
5.5	Distribution of time spent on person care, 2004.	135
6.1	Changes in the relative share of two-generation and three-generation households with children under the age of six between 1986 and 2006.	156
6.2	Labour force participation of mothers with at least one child under the age of six by type of household (1986–2006).	159
6.3	Changes in the labour force participation rate of single mothers with at least one child under the age of six (1991–2006).	161
6.4	Percentage of men and women who usually care for a family member (1991–2006).	164

6.5	Percentage of people caring for family members living in separate residence (2001–2006).	164
6.6	Percentage of caregivers for family members 65 years old and over using caring assistance.	166
7.1	Distribution of time spent on unpaid care work by sex.	180
7.2	Distribution of time spent on care of persons by sex.	181
8.1	Composition of total working time (24-hour) by sex.	200

Tables

1.1	Summary of Methodological Characteristics of Surveys	8
1.2	Female Economic Activity Rate and Share, 15+ Years, 1980, 1994, 2005	11
1.3	Summary of Results of Tobit Estimations on Unpaid Care Work	26
1.4	Summary of Results of Tobit Estimations on Care of Persons	28
2.1	Distribution of Time Spent on Activities Per Day by Sex	47
2.2	Time Spent on Paid and Unpaid Work by Age Group and Sex	52
2.3	Time Spent by Adults on Paid and Unpaid Work by Marital Status and Sex	53
2.4	Time Spent by Adults on Paid and Unpaid Work by Co-residence with Young Children and Sex	53
2.5	Time Spent by Adults on Paid and Unpaid Work by Work Status and Sex	53
2.6	Time Spent by Adults on Paid and Unpaid Work by Educational Achievement Status and Sex	55
2.7	Time Spent by Adults on Paid and Unpaid Work by Settlement Type and Sex	55
2.8	Time Spent by Adults on Paid and Unpaid Work by Household Income (Tshs 1000) and Sex	55
2.9	Time Spent on Paid and Unpaid Work by Household Composition and Sex	56

xii *Tables*

2.10	Mean Time Spent Per Day on Activities Related to Care of Persons by Sex, 24-hour Minute	60
2.11	Estimation Results on Duration of Time Spent on Care of Persons	62
2.12	Estimation Results on Duration of Time Spent on Unpaid Care Work	63
3.1	Distribution of Activities Over the Day by Sex	73
3.2	Time Spent on Paid and Unpaid Work by Population Group and Sex	75
3.3	Time Spent on Paid and Unpaid Work by Age Group and Sex	75
3.4	Time Spent on Paid and Unpaid Work by Marital Status and Sex	76
3.5	Time Spent on Paid and Unpaid Work by Child Status and Sex	77
3.6	Time Spent on Paid and Unpaid Work by Work Status and Sex	77
3.7	Time Spent on Paid and Unpaid Work by Settlement Type and Sex	78
3.8	Time Spent on Paid and Unpaid Work by Personal Income and Sex	79
3.9	Time Spent on Paid and Unpaid Work by Household Income and Sex	80
3.10	Regression Results on Duration of Time Spent on Care	85
3.11	Regression Results on Duration of Time Spent on Unpaid Care Work	85
3.12	Total Value of Unpaid Care Work and Person Care Per Year (Rbn): Different Approaches	88
4.1	Percentage Distribution of Participants in SNA and Extended SNA Activities	95
4.2	Mean Hours Spent Daily on SNA and Extended SNA by Age Group	97

Tables xiii

4.3	Mean Hours Spent Daily on Extended SNA and SNA for Individuals with Children in Their Households	99
4.4	Mean Hours Spent Daily on SNA and Unpaid Care Work by Educational Status	101
4.5	Mean Hours Spent Daily on SNA and Unpaid Care Work by Monthly Per Capita Expenditure	102
4.6	Mean Hours Spent Daily on SNA and Unpaid Care Work by Workers in Organised and Unorganised Sector	102
4.7	Mean Hours Spent Daily on Extended SNA Across Activity Classification Groups	103
4.8	Mean Hours Spent Daily on Subcategories of Unpaid Care Work	105
4.9	Mean Hours Spent Daily on Care for Sick, Disabled and Elderly	106
4.10	Mean Daily Hours Spent on Direct Child Care Activities	107
4.11	Time Spent and Participation in Direct Child Care by Demographic and Social Variables	108
4.12	Time Spent and Participation in Direct Child Care by Education and Economic Variables	110
4.13	Mean Daily Hours Spent on Subcategories of Direct Child Care	111
4.14	Time Spent and Participation in Household Maintenance by the Presence of Children in Different Age Categories	113
4.15	Mean Daily Hours Spent on Childcare-related Community Services and Help to Other Households	113
4.16	Tobit Regression Results for Time Spent on Unpaid Care Work	114
4.17	Tobit Regression Results for Time Spent on Person Care	115
5.1	Regression Outputs on Duration of Time Spent on Unpaid Care Work, 1999	123
5.2	Regression Outputs on Duration of Time Spent on Person Care, 1999	123

xiv Tables

5.3	Regression Outputs on Duration of Time Spent on Unpaid Care Work, 2004	124
5.4	Regression Outputs on Duration of Time Spent on Person Care, 2004	124
5.5	Time on Paid and Unpaid Care Work by Sex (%), 1999 and 2004	125
5.6	Time on Paid and Unpaid Care Work by Sex and Age Group (%), 1999 and 2004	127
5.7	Time on Paid and Unpaid Care Work by Sex and Education (%), 1999 and 2004	128
5.8	Time on Paid and Unpaid Care Work by Sex and Marital Status (%), 1999 and 2004	130
5.9	Time on Paid and Unpaid Care Work by Sex and Children Status (%), 1999 and 2004	131
5.10	Time on Paid Work and Unpaid Care Work by Sex and Work Status (%), 1999 and 2004	132
5.11	Time on Work and Care by Household Type (%), 1999 and 2004	133
5.12	Unpaid Care Work and Person Care as Percentage of GDP: Different Approaches	136
5.13	Total Value of Unpaid Care Work and Person Care by Year (Thousand Million Won): Different Approaches	137
5.14	Comparison of Total Annual Hours Spent on Paid Work, Unpaid Care Work and Person Care	139
6.1	Distribution of Activities Over the Day by Sex	143
6.2	Time Spent on Paid and Unpaid Work by Age Group and Sex	144
6.3	Time Spent on Paid and Unpaid Work by Marital Status and Sex	145
6.4	Time Spent on Paid and Unpaid Work by Presence of Children and Sex	145
6.5	Time Spent on Paid and Unpaid Work by Work Status and Sex	145

6.6	Time Spent on Paid and Unpaid Work by Household Income and Sex	146
6.7	Regression Results on Duration of Time Spent on Unpaid Care Work	147
6.8	Regression Results on Duration of Time Spent on Care of Persons: Males and Females Aged 15–64	149
6.9	Regression Results on Duration of Time Spent on Child Care: Co-residence with Own Child Aged Under 10	150
6.10	Twelve-country Comparison of Daily Time Use Among Married Couples with at Least One Child Aged 6 or Under	153
6.11	Trends in Daily Time Use by Mothers and Fathers with at Least One Child Under the Age of 6 (1986–2006)	155
6.12	Time Use Distribution of Fathers in Families with at Least One Child Below 6 Years of Age by Type of Household (1986–2006)	157
6.13	Time Use Distribution of Mothers in Families with at Least One Child Under the Age of 6 by Type of Household (1986–2006)	158
6.14	Time Use Distribution of Mothers with One or More Children Under the Age of 6 According to Household Type and Employment Status (1986–2006)	160
6.15	Time Use Data for Single Mothers with at Least One Child Under the Age of 6 by Type of Employment (1986–2006)	162
6.16	The Daily Time Use Distribution of Men and Women Who Provide Care for a Family Member (1991–2006)	165
6.17	The Daily Time Use Distribution of Women and Men Who Provide Care to an Elderly Family Member (or Members) According to the Use of Caring Assistance	167
7.1	Participation Rates, Mean Actor Time and Mean Population Time of the Population 15–64 Years by Sex and SNA Category	178
7.2	Participation Rates, Mean Actor Time and Mean Population Time of the Population 15–64 Years in SNA Work by Sex	179

xvi *Tables*

7.3	Participation Rates, Mean Participant Time and Mean Population Time of the Population 15–64 Years in Unpaid Care Work by Sex	179
7.4	Participation Rates and Mean Time Spent by Population 15–64 Years on Selected Activities by Area of Residence and Sex	182
7.5	Participation Rates and Mean Time Spent by Population 15–64 Years on Selected Activities by Age Group and Sex	183
7.6	Participation Rates and Mean Time Spent by Population 15–64 Years on Selected Activities by Conjugal Status and Sex	184
7.7	Participation Rates and Mean Time Spent by Population 15–64 Years on Selected Activities by Sex and Number of Children Under 6 Years in Household	185
7.8	Participation Rates and Mean Time Spent by Population 15–64 Years on Selected Activities by Activity Status and Sex	186
7.9	Participation Rates and Mean Time Spent by Population 15–64 Years on Selected Activities by Sex and Monetary Household Income Quintile	187
7.10	Care Dependency Ratio	187
7.11	Tobit Estimation of Unpaid Care Work	189
7.12	Tobit Estimation for Care of Persons	190
7.13	Estimated Value of Unpaid Care Work and Care of Persons for the Population 15–64 years, 1998 (Millions Córdobas)	192
7.14	Value of Unpaid Care Work and Care of Persons of the Population 15–64 Years Compared to Gross Domestic Product, 1998 (per cent)	192
8.1	Mean Time Spent in SNA Work, Unpaid Care Work and Care of Persons, by Sex and Age	201
8.2	Mean Time Spent in SNA Work, Unpaid Care Work and Care of Persons, by Sex and Educational Level	202
8.3	Mean Time Dpent in SNA Work, Unpaid Care Work and Care of Persons, by Sex and Labour Market Status	203
8.4	Mean Time Spent in SNA Work, Unpaid Care Work and Care of Persons, by Sex and Position in Household	204

8.5	Mean Time Spent in SNA Work, Unpaid Care Work and Care of Persons, by Sex and Type of Household	205
8.6	Mean Time Spent in SNA Work, Unpaid Care Work and Care of Persons, by Sex and Presence of Children in Household (24-hour Time)	206
8.7	Mean Time Spent in SNA Work, Unpaid Care Work and Care of Persons, by Sex and Household Absolute Poverty (24-hour Time)	207
8.8	Mean Time Per Actor and Rate of Participation in Care of Persons (%), by Sex and Age	211
8.9	Mean Time Per Actor and Participation Rate in Care of Persons (%), by Sex and Educational Level	212
8.10	Mean Time Per Actor and Participation Rate in Care of Persons (%), by Sex and Labour Market Status	212
8.11	Mean Time Per Actor and Rate of Participation in Care of Persons (%), by Sex and Position in Household	213
8.12	Mean Time Per Actor and Rate of Participation in Care of Persons (%), by Sex and Type of Household	214
8.13	Mean Time Per Actor and Participation Rate in Care of Persons (%), by Sex and Presence of Children in Household	215
8.14	Mean Time Per Actor and Participation Rate in Care of Persons (%), by Sex and Household Absolute Poverty	215
8.15	Marginal Effects for Tobit Conditional on Positive Unpaid Care Work, by Sex	217
8.16	Marginal Effects for Tobit Conditional on Positive Care of Persons, by Sex	219

Acronyms and Abbreviations

bn	billion
CSO	Central Statistical Organisation (India)
DGEyC	Dirección General de Estadística y Censos (Argentine)
EMNV	Encuesta Nacional de Medición del Nivel de Vida (Nicaragua)
ESNA	Extended System of National Accounts
GDP	Gross domestic product
ICATUS	International Classification of Activities for Time Use Surveys
ILFS	Integrated Labour Force Survey (Tanzania)
INEC	Instituto Nacional de Estadísticas y Censos (Nicaragua)
KLIP	Korean Labour and Income Panel Survey
LCTI	Long-Term Care Insurance (Japan)
LFS	Labour force survey (South Africa)
MHLW	Ministry of Health, Labour and Welfare (Japan)
MPT	Mean population time
NEA	Not economically active
NSO	National Statistics Office (Korea)
PHC	Primary health care
PR	Participation rate
R	South African rand

SC	Scheduled Caste
SNA	System of National Accounts
ST	Scheduled Tribe
STULA	Survey on Time Use and Leisure Activities (Japan)
Tshs	Tanzania shillings
TUS	Time use survey
UCW	Unpaid care work
UNDP	United Nations Development Programme
UNRISD	United Nations Research Institute for Social Development
UNSD	United Nations Statistics Division

Foreword

This volume is focused on unpaid care work—that is, the housework, care of persons and "volunteer" work performed by individuals on an unpaid basis in the homes, neighbourhoods and communities where they live. This is an area that has generally been neglected by economists (whether neoclassical or political economy) as well as by many development actors. Yet the amount of unpaid care work done, the way that the burden of the work is distributed across different individuals, and the proportion and kinds of care work that are unpaid or paid, have important implications for the well-being of individuals and households, as well as for economic dynamism and growth.

The bulk of unpaid care work across all economies and cultures is performed by women. It is therefore not surprising that feminist economists have led the call for unpaid care work to be made visible in statistics, in economic analyses and in policy making. As an important step in this direction, an increasing number of countries, including some developing countries, now collect data on how people allocate their time not only to the kind of paid work that is picked up in labour force surveys but also to other activities, both work and non-work, that are unpaid. However, the evidence is not always analysed or made accessible to a wider audience (beyond statisticians and time use specialists) nor is it used to inform policy.

This volume examines the variation across a number of countries in patterns of paid and unpaid work by gender, as well as other variables such as class and race. It is distinguished from much of the existing analysis of time use data in its focus on developing countries: five of the seven countries analysed are developing, while the sixth, the Republic of Korea, was until recently considered to be developing. The seventh country, Japan, provides an example of a highly developed country, but one with a clear gender division of labour. The volume is also timely given the growing number of policy makers, development workers, activists and academics who are interested in the issue of care, and unpaid care work in particular.

While the studies are primarily of developing countries, the volume avoids simple generalisations about developing as opposed to developed countries. It confirms that some basic facts, such as the disproportionate amount of unpaid care work performed by women, hold true across all countries, both developed and developing. However, it also reveals many differences between countries. For example, the mean time spent by Tanzanian women on work that should be "counted" (but is not) when calculating gross domestic product (GDP) is more than double that for women in South Africa, and nearly double that of Nicaraguan women. In other words, responses need to be grounded in an analysis of specific contexts, rather than assuming common patterns, which in turn strengthens the need for data collection and the type of analysis presented in this volume.

UNRISD would like to take this opportunity to thank the United Nations Development Programme (UNDP) Japan/WID Fund, the International Development Research Centre (Canada), and the Swiss Agency for Development and Cooperation (SDC) for funding the research project on Political and Social Economy of Care. As with all UNRISD projects, this work would not have been possible without core funding. We are grateful to the governments of Denmark, Finland, Mexico, South Africa, Sweden, Switzerland and the United Kingdom for their contributions.

Sarah Cook
Director, UNRISD

1 What do Time Use Studies Tell Us about Unpaid Care Work?
Evidence from Seven Countries
Debbie Budlender

INTRODUCTION

Unpaid care work—the housework and care of persons that occurs in homes and communities of all societies on an unpaid basis—is an area that has generally been neglected by economists, as well as by many development actors. This neglect is evident across virtually all schools of economics, whether neoclassical, political economy or Marxist. Yet the amount of unpaid care work done, the way that the burden of the work is distributed across different actors, and the proportion and kinds of care work that are unpaid or paid have important implications for the well-being of individuals and households, as well as for the economic growth and well-being of nations.

The bulk of unpaid care work across all economies and cultures is performed by women. It is therefore not all that surprising that feminist economists have led the call for unpaid care work to be "counted" in statistics, "accounted for" in representations of the economy, and "taken into account" in policy making (Elson 2000:21). It is also feminists who have argued that theorizing and research into welfare states and regimes need to have gender as a central focus (see Razavi 2007 for a summary of this literature).

Like the general literature on welfare states and regimes, much of the feminist work on this topic has, until now, focused on more developed countries. Similarly, until fairly recently, most of the large-scale attempts to measure unpaid work through time use surveys occurred in the more developed economies of Europe, North America and Australia. In developing countries, there were some explorations of the unpaid work of women, but these tended to be small scale, were often qualitative in nature and tended to focus on the unpaid production of goods (such as subsistence agriculture) rather than the unpaid production of services (care). Over the last decade or two an increasing number of developing countries have conducted large-scale time use surveys that provide more reliable and representative data. However, evidence of the sort presented in this book for developing countries is not widely known or available, and has not previously been presented in a way that facilitates comparison cross countries. The book is thus intended to help fill a noticeable gap in available knowledge.

Time use surveys differ from standard labour force surveys in that they ask respondents to report on all activities carried out in a specified period, such as a day or a week. In contrast, labour force surveys focus only on the forms of work that classify a person as "employed" and that are utilised in estimations of gross domestic product (GDP). Labour force surveys can therefore tell us the likelihood of a person (male or female) of a particular age or group being employed or unemployed, the type of work they do in employment and the conditions under which they work. Time use surveys, in contrast, tell us how much time an average person from a particular social group (such as male or female, young or old, rich or poor) spends on sleeping, eating, employment-related work, socializing, and unpaid care work, such as housework and caring for children, the disabled, elderly, ill and so on, in an average day or week. Time use surveys thus provide a good basis for discussing unpaid care work in more concrete terms, and for exploring how responsibility for this interacts with the performance of other activities, such as earning an income, and how it varies along a range of individual and social characteristics.

The project of the United Nations Research Institute for Social Development (UNRISD) on *Political and Social Economy of Care* aims to explore the way in which care—and in particular, care of persons—is provided by the institutions of family/household, state, market and community, and by the people within these institutions. The project has been designed to bring together the findings from in-depth quantitative and qualitative research across a range of countries so as to arrive at a nuanced understanding of the similarities and differences in care provision across different contexts.

The six "core" countries for the research project are Argentina and Nicaragua in Latin America, India and the Republic of Korea in Asia, and South Africa and Tanzania in Africa. Two countries were chosen from each of these three continents in order to have one country that was more developed, both in terms of its economy and welfare services, and another that was less so. In addition, smaller research initiatives have been conducted in Switzerland and Japan so as to include examples of care in more developed economies.

All eight countries were chosen on the basis that time use survey data were available for analysis. In the first year of the project, the research teams for each of the six core countries produced a detailed research report that analysed data from these surveys in their respective countries. A similar report was subsequently produced for Japan. Although the surveys differ in some important respects (as discussed in the following paragraph), the reports utilised a relatively similar framework and attempted to analyse similar issues. This chapter summarises and compares some of the findings from the analysis of time use data from the six core countries as well as those from Japan. The country-specific chapters that follow provide more detailed analysis of the findings in each country. However, because of space restrictions, most of the country chapters do not include all the analysis included in the reports prepared for the project. This chapter thus at times includes findings from a particular country that are not covered in the country chapter.

The socioeconomic variables used by the country teams are similar in many respects. They are, however, not always completely the same or strictly comparable. The differences between countries arise, among others, from the particular situation within each country (for example, the South African concept of race and the Indian concept of caste are not relevant for the other countries). Further differences arise because of the population covered by the surveys. These include differences in the age group covered, as well as the fact that the Argentina survey covered only the city of Buenos Aires. Further differences arise as a result of the particular instruments and methodology used for the surveys in different countries, the number and nature of days covered, the information gathered through these surveys, and the options provided for answering questions. Many of these differences are described in a paper produced for the project (Budlender 2007). Despite these differences, there is sufficient common ground to allow cross-country analysis.

This chapter consists of seven sections after this short introduction, as follows.

- *Key concepts* briefly introduces time use–related concepts utilised in later discussion in the chapter.
- *Methodologies* describes and compares some of the relevant characteristics of the methodologides used for the time use surveys in each of the seven countries.
- *Basic gender patterns* presents a set of graphs derived from standardised sex-disaggregated tables compiled for each country. These graphs give a sense of the variation in male and female levels of engagement in, and the time spent on, employment-related work, unpaid care work and care of persons more narrowly defined.
- The *Tobit estimations* reports on the econometric analysis conducted in each of the countries to determine the main factors influencing the time spent on unpaid care work and person care across the six countries.
- *Gender combined with other factors* discusses differences and similarities across countries in the way in which gender interacts with other factors explored in the Tobit estimations in determining how much care is undertaken by different individuals. In particular, it looks at how time spent differs between women and men in each of the countries in relation to the presence of young children in the household, employment status and age.
- The *care dependency ratio* presents country results for a care dependency ratio proposed by the project as an indicator of care demand, in contrast to other sections which focus primarily on the supply of care.

- *The "monetary" value of unpaid care work* discusses various approaches to assigning value to unpaid care work, and compares the results with a range of macroeconomic indicators for the six countries. These indicators include GDP, paid work, government revenue and government expenditure on social services.
- The *conclusion* offers some final remarks on the relevance of the findings.

The methodology used in the different surveys, of which the results are presented in the following section, can affect the findings. The chapter thus, of necessity, includes some technical discussion.

KEY CONCEPTS

The analysis of care in the UNRISD project, and the time use component in particular, draw on a definition of care which is, in turn, based on the System of National Accounts (SNA). The SNA is a set of internationally accepted rules for calculating GDP. These rules, in essence, define how economic growth is measured. The SNA distinguishes between "production" (or "work") and non-productive activity by defining production as any activity that one could, at least in theory, pay someone else to do. Work in a factory, as well as housework, thus constitutes production, whereas getting dressed, sleeping, socialising and studying do not.

The SNA goes further than this to distinguish production that should be included in calculations of GDP and that which should not. It states that all production of goods should be included in the calculation (in the SNA "production boundary"), whether or not the goods are sold on the market. As a result, subsistence agricultural activity, for example, would be included, as would the collection of fuel and water for household consumption. In respect of services, in contrast, only those that are sold on the market are included. Therefore, housework in one's own home, and unpaid care for children, elderly people, the ill and disabled are not included in the calculation of GDP. It is these excluded services which this book categorises as unpaid care work or "extended SNA".

Unpaid care work thus forms a key focus of this chapter, and the book as a whole. But unpaid care work can itself be disaggregated into different types of work. At a broad level, the International Classification of Activities for Time Use Surveys (ICATUS), which was used as the basis for coding in three of the seven countries, distinguishes between three sub-categories, namely (unpaid) household maintenance (broadly equivalent to housework), (unpaid) care of persons in one's own household, and (unpaid) community services and help to other households.

The UNRISD project has a special interest in care of persons, and some of the analysis that will be discussed focuses on activities that constitute such care. The classification systems of all countries covered in this book allow for care of persons to be distinguished, although in some countries the sub-categories do not cover all possible types of care of persons. Further, while the ICATUS provides explicit codes for the more passive care activities of 'supervising' children and adults in need of care, similar provision is not made in the coding systems for Nicaragua, Japan and Korea. Korea is the only country that includes a specific code for care of spouse.

In the analysis, in some cases person care is defined as equivalent to the second sub-category (that is, unpaid care of persons in one's own household). In other cases, care of persons in other households, from the third sub-category, is also considered. In practice, the inclusion of care of persons beyond the household does not substantially affect the results at the broad level presented in the following paragraphs, because care of persons in one's own household is generally far "larger" in terms of rates of participation and time spent on it than care of persons beyond the household.

A complicating factor in using an SNA–related definition is that, according to the SNA, the collection of fuel and water is considered to be production of goods, and is thus included in the production boundary. In practice, however, very few countries—and none of the six considered here—include the value of these activities when computing GDP. In addition, most people who carry out these activities would consider them part of household maintenance. The following discussion highlights, at relevant points, how the collection of fuel and water is classified. This question is obviously more important for less developed countries, where the activity is common, than it is for Japan, the Republic of Korea or the city of Buenos Aires.

In five of the countries the time use surveys were based on a *diary approach*. In this approach, respondents were asked to report what they did for each period of a 24-hour day. The periods (or "time slots") of the day used ranged from 10 minutes in the Republic of Korea to 1 hour in India and Tanzania. Whatever the period, this approach provides a full day's picture, including the time at which particular activities were undertaken. Japan used both a stylised approach, with 20 broad activities specified, for one part of the sample and a diary approach, post-coded into 62 activities, for the other part of the sample. Nicaragua used only a *stylised approach*. The Nicaragua questionnaire included 22 questions related to specific activities of the form: "Did the person spend time on family or commercial agriculture? (Yes/No)" "If yes, how much time (in hours and minutes)?" The 22 questions were followed by a further question asking about any "other activities different to those mentioned". The fieldworker was required to check that the hours and minutes totalled 24 hours, thus ensuring the full coverage of a day. Nevertheless, as noted in Budlender (2007; see also Bittman and Wajcman 2004:174), research suggests that such stylised questions produce less accurate results than a full diary.

A further potential advantage of diary-based methods is that, if designed and implemented appropriately, they are better able to capture *simultaneous activities*. This is especially important in a study of care, as care of persons—particularly "passive" care that involves supervision—is more likely than some other activities to be conducted concurrently with other activities. Ironmonger (2004:96), for example, cites Canadian data that suggest that the amount of time spent on unpaid childcare is four times as high when childcare conducted simultaneously with other activities is included. The surveys in all six countries attempted to capture simultaneous time. Argentina, South Africa and Tanzania were relatively successful in capturing simultaneous activities. In India, Japan and the Republic of Korea, respondents could name more than one activity for a particular period, but were required to rank these activities. In Argentina, South Africa and Tanzania, in contrast, simultaneous activities were given equal weight. Examination of the data reveals that relatively few simultaneous activities were recorded in India and the Republic of Korea. For Japan, the researchers did not have access to the data on "secondary" simultaneous activities and the analysis is thus confined to the "main" activities.

In Nicaragua, the prompts on specific activities previously described were followed by two further double-barrelled questions: "Did the person spend time on caring for children at the same time as other activities?" "If yes, how much time?" and "Did the person spend time on other simultaneous activities? Yes/No", "If yes, how much time?" Unfortunately, these final questions were so poorly answered that the Instituto Nacional de Estadísticas y Censos (National Institute of Statistics and Census) decided not to include them in the analysis. These data are—for the same reason—excluded from the analysis presented in this chapter. Therefore, the Nicaraguan results do not include simultaneous activities. In fact, even if the questions had been better answered, this method of asking about simultaneous activities does not identify which other activities were combined with childcare or other simultaneous activities.

Where simultaneous activities are recorded, the question arises as to what measure of duration to allocate for purposes of analysis. For example, if two activities are carried out simultaneously in a given 30-minute period, should each be allocated a period of 15 or 30 minutes? For the purposes of the analysis in the following paragraphs, the chapter distinguishes between two options. For the 24-hour minute, the available time is divided between the simultaneous activities so that all activities in a given day add up to 24 hours. The advantage of this approach is that it allows for simple comparisons of the distribution of activities over a full day, as presented, for example, in Figure 1.1.

For the "full minute", each activity is given its full duration. The advantage of this approach is that it is possible to see the full extent of time devoted to particular activities. This is particularly important in the case of an activity such as care, where performance of the activity may limit the carer in terms of what other activities can be performed at the same time, and where. In the case of Argentina, where simultaneous activities were captured to a greater

What do Time Use Studies Tell Us about Unpaid Care Work?

extent than in other countries in the sample, the full minute approach gives an average of over 28 hours per person, per day. In the case of the Republic of Korea, there was little difference in the results of the two approaches, and little analysis was carried out using the full minute approach. For Argentina, India, South Africa and Tanzania, the full minute approach was used more regularly for analysis, as deemed appropriate, although the difference between the two measures for India was small. The following discussion reports which of the two approaches is used for each type of analysis.

METHODOLOGIES

Table 1.1 summarises characteristics of the methodologies used for the country surveys that are relevant in understanding the findings and comparing findings across countries. As can be seen, all surveys analysed in this book are relatively recent, from 1999 or later. For two countries, Japan and Korea, analysis was done for surveys in two different time periods, thus allowing for some trend analysis.

The column on design establishes that a diary method was used in all countries except Nicaragua. In Nicaragua the time use information was obtained through a series of 22 questions about specific activities, as described before.

For the countries using diaries, in Japan and Korea these were mostly self-completed, while the other countries used face-to-face recall interviews. For all surveys except the one including data on Nicaragua and Questionnaire A in Japan, relatively detailed activity coding systems were used. In all these systems travel is coded separately, but according to the type of activity for which it is undertaken.

Most countries that used a diary-based method used a pre-set time period. The time period ranged from 10 minutes in Korea to 1 hour in Tanzania. Countries using longer time periods generally allowed for more than one activity to be recorded per time period—ranging from five per period for Tanzania to three per period for South Africa and Argentina, both of which used a half-hour period. India's questionnaire did not provide pre-set time periods.

The column on design further establishes that the time use survey was conducted as a stand-alone exercise in India, Japan, Korea and South Africa, while in the other countries it constituted a module of a household survey of broader scope.

The size of the samples varies widely across countries, from 1,408 individuals in Buenos Aires, Argentina to between 200,000 and 250,000 individuals in Japan. In all cases responses were weighted so as to be representative of the populatin of the relevant age group. The age group differed across countries. Tanzania had the widest age range, including all household members aged 5 years and older, while Argentina had the smallest age range, covering only those aged 15–75 years. For this chapter, analysis is

Table 1.1 Summary of Methodological Characteristics of Survey

	Design	Scope & information
Argentina	2005 Administered full 24-hour diary Post-coded Module in households survey	Buenos Aires 1,408 households 1,408 individuals 15–74 years One member per household One day
Nicaragua	1998 Administered stylised (22 categories) In household survey	2,325 households 8,756 individuals 6+ years
India	1999 Administered full 24-hour diary Post-coded Stand-alone	6 states 18,591 households 75,000 individuals 6+ years Up to three days
Korea	1999 and 2004 Self-completed 24-hour diary Post-coded Stand-alone	17,000 households 42,973 individuals 10+ years Two days
Japan	2001 and 2006 Self-completed 24-hour diary Both pre- and post-coded Stand-alone	70,000–100,000 households 200,000–250,000 individuals 15+ years Two days
South Africa	2000 Administered full 24-hour diary Post-coded Stand-alone	8,564 households 14,553 individuals 10+ years Two members per household One day
Tanzania	2006 Administered full 24-hour diary Post-coded Module in household survey	3 146 households 10,553 individuals 5+ years Seven days

restricted to those aged 15–64 years so as to allow more reliable comparisons to be made.

The number of days covered per respondent also varied. In Tanzania, each respondent was visited daily for seven consecutive days, and asked about activities done in the previous 24 hours. At the other end of the spectrum, only one day was covered for each respondent in Argentina and South Africa.

The number of respondents per household also differed across surveys. For most countries, all household members in the relevant age group were approached. However, in Argentina and South Africa one and two respondents respectively were randomly selected from members of the relevant age group.

BASIC GENDER PATTERNS

To facilitate comparison across countries, each team generated a set of age-standardised tables in relation to time spent on productive and non-productive activities, as well as time spent on the sub-categories of unpaid care work. The age group used for these tables was 15–64 years, which corresponds to the age group commonly used internationally when reporting on labour market engagement.

The following graphs and tables compare patterns across the countries in terms of three measures, namely, mean population time, participation rate and mean actor time. The *mean population time* gives the number of minutes that an "average" person in the sample spent on a particular type of activity. The *participation rate* gives the proportion of the surveyed population that was recorded as engaging in a particular type of activity. The *mean actor time* provides the number of minutes that a person spent on a particular type of activity averaged only over those who performed that activity. The mean population time is thus, in effect, a composite measure made up of the second and third measures, as "proved" by the following formula:

$$\frac{Total\ time}{Population} = \frac{Participants}{Population} \times \frac{Total\ time}{Participants}$$

Where virtually everybody undertook a particular type of activity (such as sleeping) over the period recorded in the time use survey, there is no difference between mean population time and mean actor time. Where, in contrast, only a small proportion of the population carried out a particular activity, the mean actor time might be relatively high but the mean population time relatively low as the denominator for the latter includes many people who recorded zero minutes spent on this activity. In the following figures the difference between mean population time and mean actor time is most marked for unpaid community services, for which participation rates are very low. Interpretation of all comments about greater or lesser time spent by particular groups on particular activities must thus consider which of the two time measures is at stake.

The estimates are presented separately for men and women in acknowledgement of the significant gender differences that prevail in respect of unpaid care work as well as some other types of activity.

The results presented for the seven countries must be read against the background of what has been found in previous studies which, as noted before, have focused more on developed, rather than developing, countries. They must also be read against what labour force surveys and other sources of data tell us about paid work and employment.

Elson's (2000:73–74) graphical presentation of the change in the female share of paid employment in industry and services over the period 1980–1997 reveals that the share increased or remained the same for most countries, with the most notable exceptions occurring in the transition countries of Eastern Europe. Nevertheless, in an overwhelming majority of countries, the share remained below 50 per cent. Increasing participation by women in the paid labour force should be reflected in increasing participation in SNA activities in time use surveys. One might also expect that an increased participation of women in the paid labour force would be accompanied by a decreased participation by these same women in extended SNA activities, and compensated for by increased participation by men in extended SNA. In other words, the gender division of labour in respect of SNA and extended SNA could be expected to become less stark over time.

The evidence from developed countries is mixed in this respect. Bittman, Craig and Folbre (2004:226), using Australian data covering the period 1974–1992, find that the amount of hours spent by men on childcare increased, but their share of childcare did not because the number of hours spent by women also rose over the same period. Bittman (2004) also finds that the amount of time spent by adult men on unpaid care work hardly changed over their life cycle. In contrast, Budig and Folbre (2004:52–54) suggest that the amount of time spent by women in the United States on housework has declined since 1995, and that the amount of time spent by married fathers on care increased by a small amount. Bittman et al. (2004:146–149), again using Australian data, suggest that mothers who engage in paid work do less "low-intensity" care, such as housework and supervision, but no decrease occurs in respect of "developmental" care, such as reading to and other close contact with the child. They suggest that this pattern reflects a shift in the mothers' patterns of time use closer to that of the fathers, in which "the most rewarding activities" are prioritised.

Some of the apparent contradictions in the preceding findings might be explained by differences in patterns in respect of unpaid care work as a whole and person care (or childcare, in particular) more narrowly defined. Overall, however, the evidence suggests that an increase in female engagement in paid work in developed countries has not been matched by a similarly sized increase in male engagement in unpaid care work.

The factors at work in developing countries will differ in some respects from those in more developed countries. The countries covered in this book do not exhibit substantial increases in labour force participation or in female percentage share of the labour force, at least for the period reported on by Elson. The *World's Women 1995: Trends and Statistics* includes statistics for six of the seven countries, with only Japan—which is the most developed—missing. The data are shown in Table 1.2, and suggest a few very small increases together with some larger decreases. It is only Nicaragua that records a substantial increase in both the rate of economic activity for women and women's share of the economically active. However, the estimates for 2005 as recorded in the *Human Development Report 2007–2008* record clear increases for all six countries in the subsequent period. Unfortunately, it is not possible to analyse how this might have affected time use patterns because of the absence of time use data for the earlier period. Further, Table 1.2 records the standard economic activity rate whereas Elson's observation relates to engagement in paid work. As discussed elsewhere, the two are very different measures in some of the countries covered in this book, and there might be a difference in the trends in respect of economic activity and engagement in paid work.

A further important consideration for developing countries is that the time that needs to be spent on unpaid care work will be influenced by the availability of basic services, such as safe water and electricity on site, as well as access to modern appliances. It will also be influenced by the availability—or lack of availability—of "commercial" alternatives, such as domestic workers, laundromats and ready-made meals.

The time spent on care of persons should be influenced by the proportion of the population needing care (see the following section on care dependency), the ideological or cultural emphasis placed on different types of care and—perhaps most important—the likelihood that respondents will perceive and report care as a separate activity. The latter is affected, among others, by the time use methodology used. On the ideological aspect Budig and Folbre (2004:53, 58) suggest that, in the United States, "growing social concern about the amount of time that mothers spend with their children may lead mothers to reclassify their own use of time, perceiving

Table 1.2 Female Economic Activity Rate and Share, 15+ years, 1980, 1994, 2005

	Economic activity rate (%)			Female share of economically active (%)	
Country	1980	1994	2005	1980	1994
Argentina	27	28	53	27	29
India	32	28	34	26	24
Republic of Korea	39	41	50	34	34
Nicaragua	23	30	36	22	30
South Africa	38	41	46	34	36
Tanzania	85	75	86	50	47

Source: United Nations, 1995: 143–145; United Nations Development Programme, 1007: 339–340.

care activities as more salient and therefore reporting them in more detail". They suggest further that the lesser physical effort required for housework with advances in technology might encourage respondents to report childcare as a primary activity. Smeeding and Marchand (2004:26) suggest that a reduction in family size, by decreasing other demands on the time of parents, could increase the time spent on care of children. It is also likely that where large amounts of time are needed to undertake basic household maintenance, for example, as a result of poor infrastructure and limited income, less time might be available for focused care of persons. All these factors could result in less time being recorded for care of children in less developed countries.

The temporal comparisons previously discussed for some developed countries are, unfortunately, rarely available for developing countries, as there are very few developing countries with multiple comparable time use surveys. In their absence, cross-country comparisons can reveal possible trends. Franzoni's (2005) analysis of time use data for Mexico, Nicaragua and Uruguay is a rare example of cross-country analysis of time use data from developing countries. Franzoni uses level of education as an indicator of social standing for Mexico, poverty for Nicaragua, and socioeconomic status for Uruguay. In all three countries, she finds that women of lower social standing tend to do more preparation of meals but less childcare than those with higher standing. To the extent that "development" results in higher overall social standing of a country's inhabitants, related changes in patterns of time use over time might be found as a country "develops".

The SNA–Related Categories

Figure 1.1 shows the patterns across the three major categories into which all activities can be divided, namely SNA, extended SNA and non-productive activities. The first includes all activities that should be included when calculating a country's GDP because they fall within the narrow production boundary of the SNA. The second category is equivalent to unpaid care work and represents all activities that are recognised in the SNA as production or work, but are not included when calculating GDP. The final category encompasses all those activities that are not considered to be work.

As expected, across all countries, and across both male and female, 100 per cent of the population does some non-productive activity. In particular, virtually all people will sleep or eat in any 24-hour period. A further constant across all countries is that among women, participation rates are higher in respect of extended SNA than for SNA proper. For most countries, there is a large difference in female participation rates between these two categories. The exception is Tanzania, where the participation rate for SNA is 96 per cent, and there is thus inadequate "space" for a large difference between this and extended SNA. Although, as explained in the next paragraph, the Tanzanian participation rates are biased upward compared to those of other countries, as a result of the methodology, the high SNA rates also reflect the fact that in 2006, 89.6 per cent of the population aged 15 years and older was recorded as economically active, with rates of 90.5 per cent for males and 88.8 per cent for females (Meena 2007).

Tanzania has by far the highest female rates of participation in SNA work, followed by India. The Tanzanian pattern is partly explained by the fact that Tanzania's participation rate represents participation recorded over a seven-day period, whereas for other countries only one or two days of activities were recorded for each person. Increasing the number of days increases the chances of a person undertaking a particular activity. A proxy one-day participation rate for Tanzania, obtained by treating each person-day as a separate observation, yields a female participation rate of 83 per cent in SNA activities and 94 per cent for extended SNA.

SNA work is not necessarily equivalent to paid work. In Tanzania, for example, 71.7 per cent of employed females work on their own farm or *shamba*, and many of these are subsistence farmers (Meena 2007). Further, in India, South Africa and Tanzania collection of fuel and water was included under SNA work despite the fact that it is not included in the estimation of GDP. The very low rate of female SNA participation for Nicaragua can thus be partly explained by the fact that the collection of fuel and water was considered part of unpaid care work for this country. The relatively low rate for South Africa despite the inclusion of fuel and water collection reflects the low employment (and high unemployment) rates for both women and men. In September 2000, for example, the employment

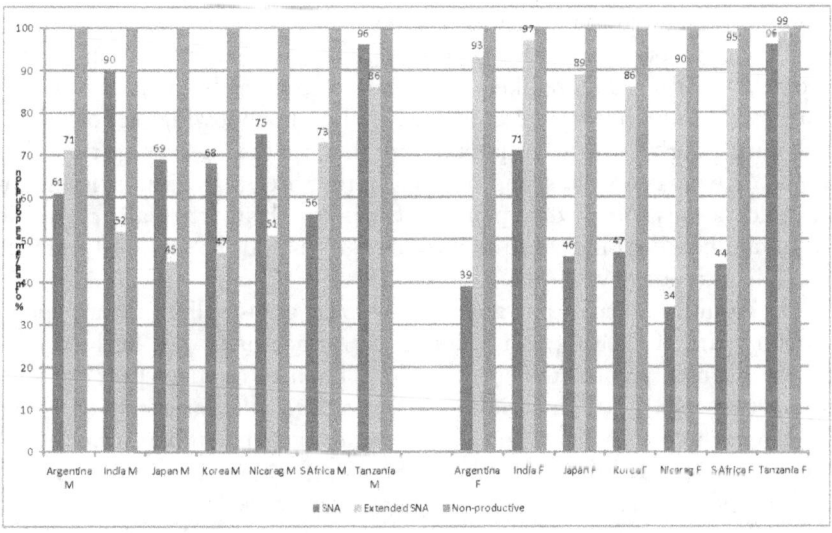

Figure 1.1 Participation rates by SNA category, country and sex.

rate for South African women aged 15 years and older was 48.6 per cent (author's calculations and labour force survey data).

There is far less variation among women in the countries included in the survey in respect of participation in extended SNA work. Engagement is lowest in the Republic of Korea, at 86 per cent. The fact that Japan and Nicaragua have very similar rates suggests that level of development is not a major determinant of participation.

For men, the participation rate in SNA work is higher than in extended SNA for five countries (India, Japan, the Republic of Korea, Nicaragua and Tanzania), but lower in the remaining two. The difference in the male participation rates in SNA and extended SNA work is largest for India, although a similarly large gap in the reverse direction is not found for Indian women. The two countries—Argentina and South Africa—for which the pattern is reversed (that is, male SNA is lower than male extended SNA) have the lowest male SNA participation rates, while male participation in unpaid care work is not particularly high when compared to the other countries. For South Africa, the low rate for male SNA is explained by the high unemployment rates in the country.

For all countries except Tanzania, the SNA participation rate is noticeably higher for men than women. Tanzania's "exceptionalism" remains even if we use the one-day proxy described previously. For all countries the extended SNA participation rate is noticeably higher for women than men. The gender gap in participation is larger in respect of extended SNA than in SNA across all countries. This is somewhat similar to the findings for developed countries reported before, where female engagement in paid work tends to converge more to male engagement, while the reverse does not occur in respect of male engagement in unpaid care work. A crude interpretation of these patterns is that, using this measure, women are more likely than men to work across all countries if all types of work are considered, and that women are more likely than men to combine both types of work. Further evidence in this respect is presented in the following section.

Figure 1.2 gives the mean population time, that is the average time that a man or woman would spend on each of the three activities, including in the calculations those who spend no time. For this particular graph, the mean number of minutes for the three categories adds up to 1,440 which is equivalent to one day.

The figure confirms that men and women across all countries spend a major part of each day on non-productive activities. For both women and men, India records the smallest proportion of the day spent on non-productive activities, while South Africa records the largest proportion. Within each country, men and women tend to spend similar amounts of time on non-productive activities. For South Africa, the high proportion of the day spent on non-productive activities mirrors the fact that the country also reports the shortest proportion of time spent on SNA activities. This, in turn, reflects the high unemployment rates in the country. For India,

What do Time Use Studies Tell Us about Unpaid Care Work? 15

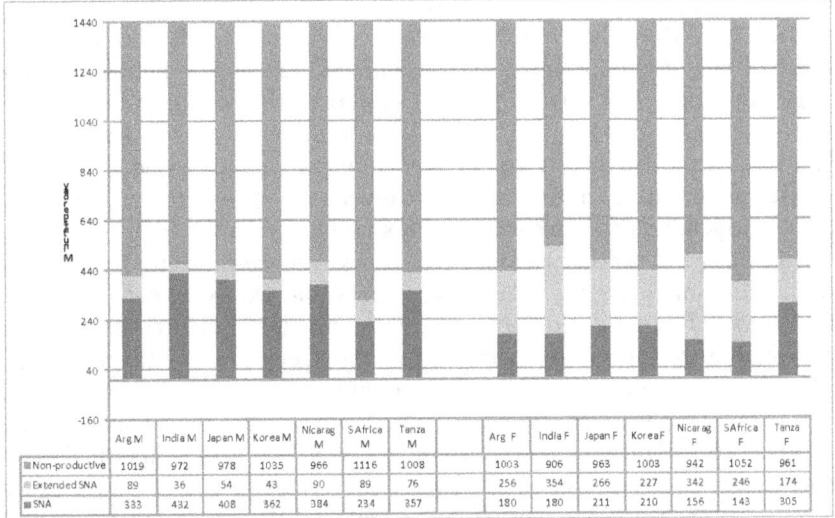

Figure 1.2 Mean time spent per day on activities by SNA category, country and sex for full sample population.

the relatively small amount of time spent on non-productive work reflects particularly high times recorded for men on SNA work, and high times for women on extended SNA.

Where there is a male–female difference, women tend to spend less time than men on non-productive activities. The converse is that women tend to spend more time working than men do, if all types of work are considered. Pacholok and Gauthier (2004:211) report a similar pattern for Canada and Germany, but find that in Sweden men tend to spend more time than women on paid and unpaid work combined. Similarly, in a larger sample of 27 "high human development" and six "medium and low human development" countries listed in the 2007/2008 *Human Development Report*, only three—the Netherlands, Norway and Sweden—report longer combined hours on SNA and expanded SNA for men than women (UNDP 2007:342).

While non-productive activity consumes the largest proportion of people's time, extended SNA accounts for the least time of the three categories for men across countries, and the least time for women in one country—Tanzania. As previously noted, much of the SNA work of Tanzanian women would be unpaid, including the collection of fuel and water.

Figure 1.2 clearly shows that women tend to spend more time on unpaid care work than men. For all countries, the mean time for women is more than twice that for men. The gender gap is most marked in India, where women spend nearly 10 times as much time on extended SNA work than men. The mean time for Indian women is about double that for Tanzanian women. Men from the three Asian countries, India, Japan and the Republic of Korea, tend to do noticeably less unpaid care work than men in the other countries. The gap for India is similar to that reported by Bittman and Wajcman (2004:178) for "'familistically' oriented" Italy, while that for Tanzania is similar to that for "gender equity conscious" Sweden.

Men tend to spend more time than women on SNA work across all countries. The gender difference is relatively small in Tanzania. In India, in contrast, men spend nearly two and a half times as much time on SNA work as women do, mirroring the much longer times that women spend on unpaid care work. Thus, while the previous graph suggested high rates of participation in SNA work for Indian women, the time spent is not particularly high. The patterns accord with those for economic activity of females aged 15 years and older as a percentage of male activity, where the Tanzanian percentage is the highest for the six countries, at 97 per cent, while the Indian percentage is second lowest, at 42 per cent (the percentage for Nicaragua is even lower, at 41 per cent) (UNDP 2007:338ff). The mean time spent by Tanzanian women on SNA work is more than double that for women in South Africa, and nearly double that of Nicaragua. South African men record the shortest mean times for SNA work, while Indian men record the longest average times. As before, the South African pattern reflects the high unemployment rates. Conversely, the Indian pattern reflects high employment rates and long hours of work.

Figure 1.3 shows the mean time spent by actors on each of the SNA–related activity types. There is no change in the time spent on non-productive activities, as these had participation rates of 100 per cent. The bars for non-productive activities are nevertheless included to allow comparison with the time spent on the other two categories. For SNA and extended SNA, the actor times are by definition longer than the population mean times. Further, because men tend to have higher participation rates in SNA–related activities, the difference between mean population time and mean actor time on these activities is greater for women than it is for men. The opposite gender pattern holds in respect of extended SNA activities, that is, the difference between mean population time and mean actor time is greater here for men than for women. All of this results in smaller apparent gender gaps for mean actor time than for mean population time. For Argentina, for example, the mean population time spent on unpaid care work for men is 35 per cent that of women's time, while the mean actor time is 45 per cent that of women's time.

As with mean population time, the mean actor time spent by men on SNA activity exceeds that spent on extended SNA activity across all countries. The difference is largest for Japan and smallest for Tanzania.

For women, the focus on mean actor time results in a reversal of the pattern in Figure 1.2 in respect to time spent on SNA and extended SNA activities in all countries but India. This pattern is explained by the fact

What do Time Use Studies Tell Us about Unpaid Care Work? 17

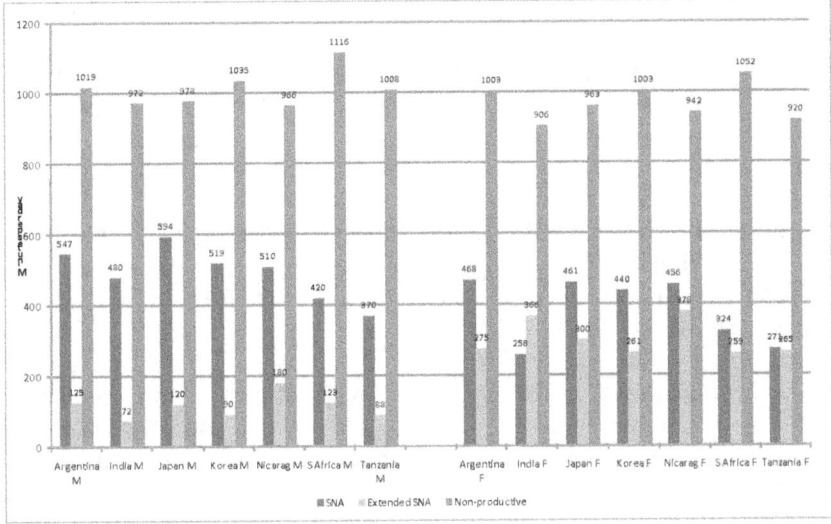

Figure 1.3 Mean time spent per day on activities by SNA category, country and sex for actors.

that the bars refer to different groupings of women. Thus the longer times are recorded for relatively small numbers of women engaged in SNA work, while the shorter times are recorded for relatively larger numbers of women engaged in extended SNA work.

Perhaps the most important message from the actor means is that population means can obscure the fact that within groups which overall engage very little in a particular type of activity, some individuals might spend extensive time on it. Conversely, high actor means can obscure the fact that only some individuals may be engaging intensely in a particular activity while the majority do very little or do not engage at all. The following discussion of distribution patterns highlights the differences between women and men in this respect.

This section concludes with a graph (Figure 1.4) that provides a simple comparison of the volume of SNA and extended SNA work done in each country. The comparison differs from that presented in Figure 1.2 in that the average hours per individual male/female are multiplied by the size of the male and female population aged 15–64 years.

The size of both the population and the economy varies enormously across the six countries, and a graphic comparison in absolute volume of hours is therefore not sensible. Instead, the data are standardised across the countries by assuming that all hours spent on SNA work and unpaid care work in a particular country constitute 100 per cent of the full economy. The percentage of this total volume that constitutes SNA and unpaid care work performed by women and men is then calculated. Thus the percentages shown in the bars for Argentina demonstrate that 23 per cent of all hours of work performed by the population aged 15–64 in the city of Buenos Aires consist of SNA work done by women, 35 per cent of the hours consist of SNA work done by men, and 32 per cent and 9 per cent are accounted for by hours of extended SNA work done by women and men respectively.

Figure 1.4 shows marked variation among countries in terms of both relative size of the SNA and unpaid care work components and the sex composition of each component. This chapter focuses first on the first aspect, namely the relative "size" of SNA and unpaid care work in the different countries.

In Nicaragua and South Africa, the SNA and unpaid care work components are almost equal in size. In all the other countries, the SNA component is noticeably larger than the unpaid care work component. In Argentina, Japan and the Republic of Korea, this pattern could reflect commercialisation of care services. In Tanzania, the predominance of SNA work reflects the small proportion of time spent by both women and men on unpaid care work, and high levels of engagement in SNA work. In India it is caused, among others, by the very long hours on SNA work recorded for men. Alternatively, if Nicaragua and South Africa are taken as exceptions, the relatively low amount of SNA work could be partly explained by high unemployment rates.

Earlier estimates of the division of total work time between SNA and non–SNA for several developing and developed countries show a similar wide range (UNDP 1995:91). For developing countries (covering urban areas of six countries, rural areas of five countries, and combined areas of one country), on average SNA work accounted for 54 per cent of total work time. However, the SNA percentage ranged from 45 per cent for the Republic of Korea in 1990 to 73 per cent in the Philippines in 1975–1977. For 13 developed countries, on average SNA work accounted for 49 per cent of total work time and ranged from 35 per cent in the Netherlands in 1987 to 68 per cent in Denmark in 1987. With the exception of these two outliers, the SNA percentage for all remaining developed countries lay between 44 per cent and 52 per cent.

The earlier estimates are probably less reliable than those for the seven countries studied here because of a greater variation in methodology, with some of the samples being small, and some data sources dating from the 1970s. In addition, for developing countries the estimates were often reported separately for urban and rural areas, and sometimes only for one of these. Nevertheless, the figures suggest that the extent of the dominance of SNA work in the Japan, Republic of Korea, Tanzania and India is unusual.

In terms of sex composition, all countries have, as expected, more hours spent by men on SNA work and by women on unpaid care work. Male dominance with SNA work is, however, much more marked in India and Nicaragua than in other countries and least marked for the city of Buenos Aires and South Africa. The larger number of women doing unpaid care work is most marked in India, and far less obvious in Tanzania. In terms of overall sex division, if all work is included, South Africa stands at one extreme, with men's volume of work equivalent to only 74 per cent of the volume performed by women. India stands at the other extreme, with men's work equivalent to 94 per cent of the volume attributable to women.

The Components of Unpaid Care Work

The previous sub-section focused on three major divisions into which activities can be categorised, namely SNA, extended SNA and non-productive activities. This section examines the second division—extended SNA or unpaid care work—in more detail. For purposes of analysis a three-way (sub-)categorisation is used, namely, household maintenance, unpaid care for persons in the household, and unpaid community services and help to other households (care for persons beyond the household, or unpaid community services). This finer disaggregation of the three main categories helps explore the extent to which the differing patterns found for developed countries in respect of unpaid care work in general, and person care in particular, are replicated in developing countries. It also helps explore whether the level of development might affect the amount of time spent on care of persons.

In the previous sub-section, the analysis was carried out in terms of 24-hour minutes so that the mean population time would add up neatly

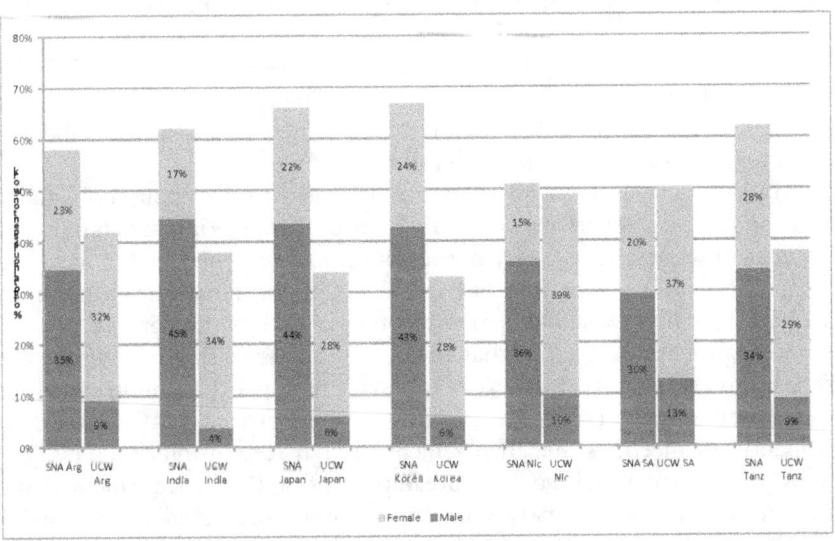

Figure 1.4 Composition of hours spent on SNA and unpaid care work by sex.

to 24 hours. In this sub-section, full minutes are used for those countries (Argentina, India, South Africa, Tanzania) where the recording of simultaneous activity allowed this distinction. Full minutes are the preferred measure here, as evidence from other countries (see, for example, Ironmonger 2004) has revealed that care of persons is especially likely to be done simultaneously with other activities. Further, person care tends to be reported as a secondary rather than main activity when performed in conjunction with other activities.

Figure 1.5 shows the participation rates for men and women across the countries. Participation rates in household maintenance are markedly higher than for the other sub-categories for both men and women across all countries. Participation rates in unpaid community services are lower than for all other sub-categories for both men and women in these countries. The gap between participation in person care and unpaid community services is generally large, with the exceptions of Tanzania and for men in South Africa. In Tanzania, the participation rate for unpaid community services is noticeably higher for both men and women than in all other countries. This is a result of the methodology used rather than any real difference in engagement in unpaid community services as time spent being interviewed for the time use survey was interpreted as an unpaid contribution to the community and given an activity code in this sub-category. If participation in the time use survey is excluded, Tanzanian participation rates in unpaid community services fall to 2 per cent for men and 4 per cent for women. This is very similar to the patterns found in other countries.

The second exceptional case where there is a relatively small gap between participation in the care of individuals and unpaid community services involves South African men. Here the explanation is that very few South African men engage in either of these sub-categories of activities.

The relatively low participation rates in care of persons for both men and women in Japan could, at least in part, be a result of the activity coding system used, which provided only one code—"help to a family member"—for care of persons other than babies and children.

Women are far more likely than men to engage in both household maintenance and care of persons across all the countries. For unpaid community services, in contrast, levels of participation are very similar for men and women, except in Argentina. The fact that the Argentine rates for women are relatively high when compared to other countries (except Tanzania) is especially interesting, given that the survey in Argentina excluded some activity codes for this sub-category that were used in other countries. These were community work, such as cooking for collective celebration, and participation in meetings and involvement in civil responsibilities. The high rates seem to accord with a widespread perception that Latin America, and Argentina in particular, have very active community-based and voluntary sectors, and that women tend to be especially active in these sectors (Jelin 1990). However, half of the unpaid community care services recorded for

What do Time Use Studies Tell Us about Unpaid Care Work? 21

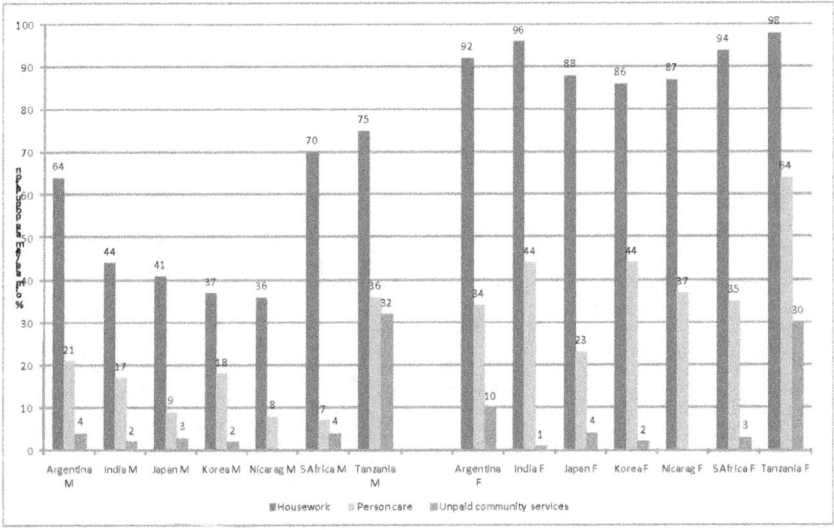

Figure 1.5 Participation rates by sub-category of unpaid care work, country and sex.

Argentine represent care of children outside the household rather than other forms of community engagement. The exclusion of participation in meetings could account for the unusual gender pattern in that men are probably more likely than women to attend meetings.

The fact that men's performance relative to that of women is "best" in respect of unpaid community services could constitute yet another reflection of the public-private divide, in that men might be more open to participating in unpaid care work when it is in a more public sphere.

Figure 1.6 shows the mean time spent on the different sub-categories of unpaid care work. The clearest message from this graph is that women tend to spend substantially more time than men on both household maintenance and care of persons across all countries. The gender gap is largest for India and Tanzania in respect of household maintenance, and smallest for South Africa. In India, where there is also a large gender gap for unpaid care work more generally, men do less than a tenth of the amount of housework done by women. The smaller gap for South Africa could reflect the diverse household and family composition and lower marriage rates than in other countries. This could mean that fewer men are able to rely on women partners to do housework for them.

The gender gap in respect of care of persons, in contrast, is largest for South Africa and smallest for Argentina. In South Africa, men do just over a tenth of the amount of person care carried out by women. The South African pattern could perhaps again be partly explained by the fractured

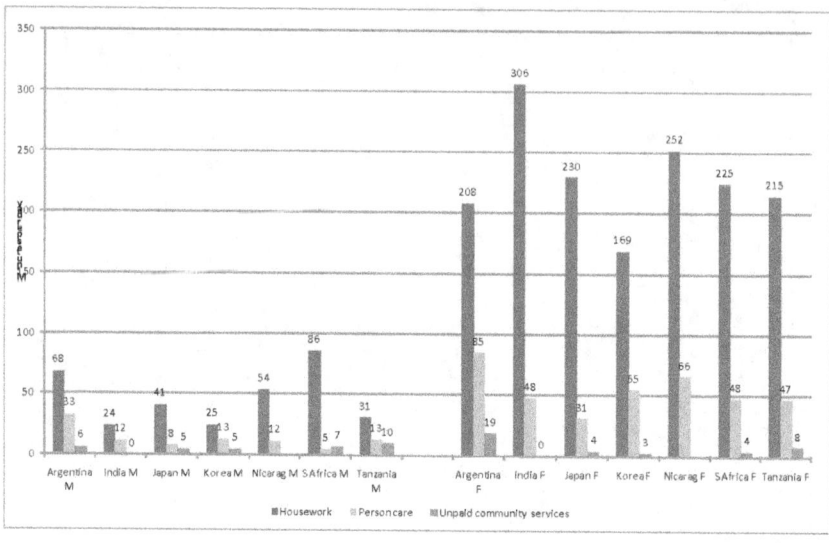

Figure 1.6 Mean time spent per day on activities by sub-category of unpaid care work, country and sex for full sample population.

family set-up, where fewer than half of all children live with their fathers and many adults do not live with their partners.

The relatively small amounts of time spent on care of persons accord with findings for more developed countries. In the 2007/2008 *Human Development Report*, only two (Ireland and Finland) of the 27 high human development countries, and one (Nicaragua) of the six medium and low human development countries, record an average of more than 1 hour per day on care of children for women aged 20 to 74 years. For men, the same two high human development countries are again the only ones reporting more than 20 minutes per day, while this situation is not found in any of the less developed countries (UNDP 2007:342). The relatively small amounts of time are, in part, a reflection of the fact that a much smaller proportion of the population engages in care of persons than in housework. This results in reduced means for care of persons. The small amounts of time could also reflect under-reporting of care of persons, particularly where this work is done simultaneously with other activities and does not involve direct physical interaction with the person being cared for.

For unpaid community services it is difficult to comment, beyond noting the very small amounts of time recorded across all countries. The definition and understanding of unpaid community services probably also differs more across countries than that of care of persons or housework. In the case of India, the low participation rates combined with relatively small amounts of time results in a mean close to zero minutes.

What do Time Use Studies Tell Us about Unpaid Care Work? 23

The higher amounts for Tanzania have been explained previously. If participation in the time use survey is excluded, the means fall to three minutes for men and two minutes for women. Argentine women thus become the real exception, with their record of 19 minutes per day across the population.

Figure 1.7 presents the mean actor time for the three sub-categories of unpaid care work. As previously noted, the mean actor times tend to reduce gender and other gaps when compared with mean population times. The graph still shows women spending more time than men on both household maintenance and care of persons across countries. The relative gender difference is, as expected, much smaller than before. It is, however, still very marked, particularly for Tanzania in respect of household maintenance. Comparing across countries, Indian women who engage in this activity— and 96 per cent of them do—far outclass all other groups in the amount of time spent on housework. This could partly reflect less developed infrastructure, although the collection of fuel and water is not classified as part of unpaid care work for India.

For unpaid community services, men record longer times than women in all countries except Argentina. (The estimates, after excluding time spent responding to the time use survey, would be 44 minutes for men and 28 for women in Tanzania.) The gender difference in time spent on unpaid community services is particularly noticeable in the Republic of Korea.

The graphs presented in this section have shown the cross-country gender patterns in respect of the three SNA categories, and the three sub-categories of unpaid care work.

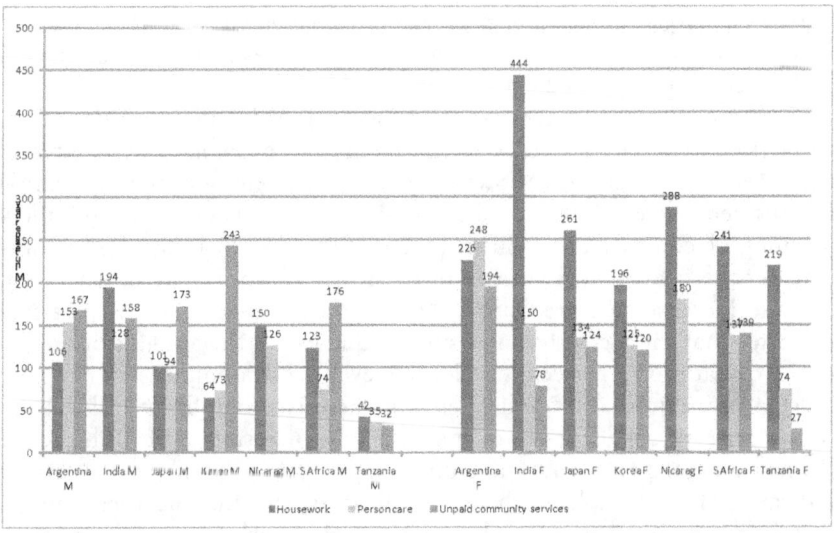

Figure 1.7 Mean time spent per day on sub-categories of unpaid care work by country and sex for actors.

THE TOBIT ESTIMATIONS

The Tobit estimations discussed in this section explore which factors beyond gender influence the time spent on unpaid care work and care of persons in different countries, as well as the direction of their influence (whether a factor tends to increase or decrease the amount of time spent on care). Subsequently, the chapter explores the way in which gender and three of the variables available for all countries—age, employment status and having children in the household—interact.

The Tobit estimations, like other regressions, make it possible to separate out the influence of different factors on the amount of care undertaken. This is especially important in situations where one factor is itself dependent on another factor. For example, a simple tabulation by age would show a clear pattern of increased engagement in, and time spent on, care of persons with increasing age. In reality, however, part of this pattern could be explained by the fact that older people are more likely to be married, and more likely to have children, with both of these characteristics in and of themselves tending to result in increased engagement in the care of persons. The Tobit estimation thus, in effect, "controls" for each of the other factors included in the estimation when calculating whether, and to what extent, a factor is influential.

The Tobit estimation method is especially designed for situations where the data are "censored" at one or either end. This makes the method particularly appropriate for time use data where the values are censored at value zero because an individual cannot spend less than zero minutes in a day on any activity. The records with zero values are included in the estimations. (The Argentina chapter presents marginal values that are calculated only in respect of observations with non-zero values.) The estimations are performed on unweighted data.

Table 1.3 summarises the results of the Tobit estimations performed for the various country datasets. It includes only those factors that were tested for at least two countries. Showing the relative strength of the association for different factors for each of the countries in a way that would allow meaningful comparison is difficult, and the table therefore shows only whether the factor has a positive or negative influence, that is, whether it tends to increase or decrease the amount of care undertaken. A plus sign indicates that the factor has a positive influence on the amount of unpaid care work at the 95 per cent confidence level, while a minus sign indicates a negative influence. "Y" indicates that there is a significant influence at the 95 per cent confidence level, but either the direction of the influence or the nature of the factor are too complicated to allow simple plus or minus indicators. For example, with some indicators, the amount of care might first increase and then fall, while with factors such as family structure, more than a binary choice (such as male/female) is involved. The letters "ns" indicates that the factor was tested but not found to be significant at this level. A cell left blank indicates that the factor was not included in the Tobit estimation. For the purposes of assigning plus or minus in respect of race and caste, white (in South Africa) is considered higher status than other races, and special caste (in India) lower status than others.

For several factors, the results are fairly consistent across countries. As expected, being male tends to result in doing less unpaid care work across all countries. This factor has the greatest influence (largest coefficient in absolute terms) of all tested factors in all countries except Argentina. In Argentina, being male is the second strongest factor, after being a spouse/partner. For all countries, having a (young) child in the household tends to increase the amount of unpaid care work done. The coefficient for age is always positive, while that for age squared is negative. This suggests an initial increase in the amount of unpaid care work performed with increasing age, followed by a decrease. The strength of this association will vary according to the age range covered for the estimation.

Where the influence of household and individual income or expenditure were tested and a significant association found, the amount of unpaid care work tended to decrease with increases in income. This could be explained by several factors, including the poorer infrastructure and technology available to poor households, less ability to buy paid care and larger household size.

Being employed tends to decrease the amount of unpaid care work carried out in all countries except Tanzania, where employed people were inclined to do more unpaid care work. The difference may be partly explained by the very high employment rate for adults in Tanzania. For most countries, being married tends to increase the amount of unpaid care work done.

For the developed countries that they examine, Pacholok and Gauthier find that women's engagement in housework tends to decrease as the level of education increases (2004:199). In the present study, the influence of education differs across countries, and sometimes across levels of education in a particular country (that is, there is a non-linear relationship). In Japan and South Africa, the amount of unpaid care work is likely to increase with the level of education. In the Republic of Korea, those with a middle level of education tend to do less unpaid care work than those with lower or higher levels, while in Tanzania the pattern is reversed, in that those with no schooling or with secondary education and above do less than those with primary education. In India, the association with education is not statistically significant. The cross-country comparisons are complicated by the different levels of education prevailing in a country. Thus, "middle level" for the Republic of Korea means something very different to "middle level" for Tanzania. The comparisons are further complicated by the fact that some countries used categories (discrete variables) for the estimation, while others used a continuous variable.

Table 1.4 presents the results for the Tobit estimation in respect of care of persons. In this case, having a young child in the household is the strongest

Table 1.3 Summary of Results of Tobit Estimations on Unpaid Care Work

	Argentina	India	Japan	Korea	Nicaragua	S. Africa	Tanzania
Male	-	-	-	-	-	-	-
Employed	-	-	-	-		-	+
Age	+	+	+	+	+	+	+
Age squared	-	-	-	-	-	-	-
Child in household	+	+	+	+	+	+	+
Education	ns	ns	+	Y	+	+	Y
Married	+	+	+	+	+	ns	+
Household income/ expenditure	+	ns			-	-	-
Caste/race		-				-	
Rural		-			+		-

factor across all countries except Nicaragua. The association with children might have been muted in Nicaragua because the presence of children up to age 18 was used, while a younger cut-off point was used in most other countries. Again, being male again tends to result in less care work being done. The pattern in respect of age is similar to that for unpaid care work. However, age is not significant for Nicaragua, neither age nor age squared is significant for Japan, and the coefficients for age squared are very close to zero for some of the other countries. The Nicaraguan and Japanese exceptionalism here is probably explained by the fact that a separate factor, being a child (aged 6–17 years), was also included in the estimation for Nicaragua, while a separate factor for being old was included for Japan.

Being married tends to increase the amount of care of persons, even in South Africa, where this factor was not significant for unpaid care work. The pattern in respect of education still varies, with less care of persons being done by the more educated in India and Tanzania, but more in the Republic of Korea and South Africa. In Japan, those with lower and higher levels of education do more care of persons than those with middle level. Tanzania is again an exception in terms of employment, with more person care being done in Tanzania by those who are employed but less in other countries.

Where household income is found to be influential, those who are poor tend to undertake more care of persons in Tanzania, but less in India. This factor is, however, not found to be significant in Argentina, Japan or South Africa. And personal income is not found to be significant in Argentina, despite being significant for unpaid care work. Race (in South Africa), caste (in India) and rural residence (in Tanzania) are no longer significant, but living in rural areas tends to result in a decrease in care of persons in India and Nicaragua.

While the Tobit estimations provide some support for the hypothesis that, within countries, the amount of unpaid care work decreases with income and status, they do not provide clear support for the hypothesis that the amount of person care also decreases with income or status.

GENDER COMBINED WITH OTHER FACTORS

As previously noted, the Tobit estimation "controls" for each of the other factors included in the estimation when calculating whether, and to what extent, a factor is influential. It thus shows the relative strength of each factor. What the Tobit estimations presented before do not show clearly, however, is how the patterns for male and female might differ in respect of each of the other factors. (The chapter on Japan includes separate male and female Tobit estimations that explore this aspect.) This section draws out some of the patterns emerging from the tabulations presented in the country papers in respect of participation rates and means. It focuses on

Table 1.4 Summary of Results of Tobit Estimations on Care of Persons

	Argentina	India	Japan	Korea	Nicaragua	S. Africa	Tanzania
Male	-	-	-	-	-	-	-
Employed	ns	-					+
Age	+	+	ns	+	ns	+	+
Age squared	-	-	ns	-	-	-	-
Childed	+	+	+	+	+	+	+
Education	ns	-	Y	+	+	+	-
Married		+	+	+	+	+	+
Household income	ns	+	Y		ns	ns	-
Caste/race		ns				ns	
Rural		-			-		ns

the factors that were tested for virtually all countries and shown before to be influential across most of the countries: age, employment and having a child in the household. The discussion focuses on unpaid care work rather than care of persons, but for the most part the patterns in respect of care of persons are very similar to those for unpaid care work as a whole.

Age

For all countries, men and women in the "middle" age groups (typically 18–45 years, or a smaller sub-group) are more likely to engage in SNA work, and tend to spend longer on it. Across all countries adult males were more likely than adult females to engage in SNA work and also more likely to spend more time on this work. While the Nicaraguan team pinpointed the 18–30 year age group as the one with the greatest gender difference in participation in SNA and paid work, it also noted a sharper fall off in engagement in SNA work for older women than older men. A similar pattern is likely in other countries. In India, older urban women (aged 46–64) who did SNA work tended to spend more time on it than the younger women did. In some countries (the Republic of Korea and Tanzania), the strong overall gender pattern in respect of SNA work did not hold for children.

For most countries, the middle age groups of both women and men were also more likely to perform unpaid care work than those of other age groups. In Nicaragua, however, participation rates in unpaid care work were highest for men among those who are 50 years or older. While Nicaraguan women's rates declined somewhat with age, they were still twice as likely as men to perform unpaid care work. In Argentina, hours spent on unpaid domestic work for those who engaged in it tended to be longer for older people, especially among women. In India, a similar pattern was found for older men in respect of unpaid care work more generally. In Nicaragua there was little variance with age in the time spent by women and men on unpaid care. In South Africa and Tanzania, there was little difference across age groups in the male mean population time spent on unpaid care work. Young South African girls were three times as likely to do unpaid care work as young boys.

Presence of Children in the Household

In almost all countries, there were indications that engagement in unpaid care work, as well as direct care of persons, was more intense when there were children in the household, and decreased as the age of the youngest child increased. Nevertheless, women were always far more likely than men to do this work. Further, while the pattern of increased engagement in unpaid care work held across all countries for women, this was not the case for men. Thus in India, men in households with no children spent the most time on extended SNA, while the age of the child in households with children had no noticeable effect on men's engagement in this work. Similarly, in Nicaragua, South Africa and Tanzania, the time spent by men on unpaid care work stayed more or less constant when there were children in the household.

In Argentina, South Africa and Tanzania, women with young children in the household were not noticeably less likely than other women to engage in SNA work. In South Africa, women with children in the household were more likely than others to do SNA work, although women with young children were less likely to engage than those with older children. This pattern could reflect the greater likelihood of mothers and their children living apart from the children's father, forcing the mother to provide both financial and other care to the children. In Tanzania, the SNA work performed by women with young children was less likely to be paid than the work done by those living without children. This could, at least in part, reflect the greater presence of children in rural areas, where unpaid SNA work is very common.

In strong contrast to the aforementioned countries, women with young children in India, Japan, the Republic of Korea and Nicaragua were less likely to engage in, and spent less time on, SNA work. In Japan, the Republic of Korea, Nicaragua and South Africa, men living with preschool children were far more likely than others to engage in SNA work, although the time spent on this work was not always longer than for other employed men. In Tanzania, the same trend was found, but was not as strong as in the other countries, perhaps because of the overall high rates of engagement in SNA work. In South Africa, 9–10 per cent of men with young children living with them did both paid work and care of persons in the previous 24 hours, while this was the case for 19 per cent of women with young children.

Employment

Strictly speaking, work status distinguishes between three situations—employed, unemployed and not economically active. The unemployed are those who are not doing SNA work but would like to do so, while the not economically active are those who do not want to, or are unable to, work. The most common reasons offered for the not economically active status are that the person is a full-time student, full-time homemaker, ill or disabled, or too old to work. In the country papers, the unemployed groupings were often very small, especially when analysis was restricted to adults. The unemployed and not economically active are thus combined in the following analysis, with the main distinction being between those who are employed and those who are not.

By definition, both women and men who are employed are expected to have higher rates of engagement in SNA work than those who are not employed. One might even expect an exact match between work status and engagement (or not) in SNA activities. There are several reasons why the match is not perfect. First, the collection of fuel and water in most countries does not classify a person as employed even though it is, strictly speaking, an SNA activity. Second, the diary day used for the time use survey, in most cases, fell outside the reference period used to classify a person as employed or not employed. Third, the standard survey questions may not fully capture all forms of labour force engagement.

In all countries where employment was considered, employed women were less likely to do unpaid care work than those who were not employed. In India, this pattern was stronger in respect of urban than rural women. Nevertheless, across all countries, employed women still had very high participation rates in this form of work.

In Argentina, employed men were more likely to do unpaid care work than those not employed. In India and Nicaragua, the opposite pattern held. In the Republic of Korea, employed men were less likely to do unpaid care work in 1999, but by 2004 this trend was no longer evident. In South Africa and Tanzania, unemployed men did more unpaid care work than those who were employed, but those not economically active did the least. However, employed men undertook more care of persons than unemployed men. These contrasting patterns for South Africa and Tanzania could be partly explained by age factors, in that those who are slightly older are also more likely to be employed and to have children.

This relatively short section highlights the fact that even where general patterns in respect of individual factors influencing the amount of care work carried out are similar across countries, there could be substantial differences among countries in how these factors operate in respect of women and men. These differences include the direction of influence (that is, whether the amount of unpaid care work tends to increase and fall) and the strength of the influence. In general, the factors tend to have a greater effect on women than on men, with men's patterns varying less with life cycle.

THE CARE DEPENDENCY RATIO

The fact that the presence of children in the household tends to result in respondents taking on more unpaid care work and more care of persons calls for discussion of the "demand" for care within and across countries relative to the potential supply. This is done by developing a proxy "care dependency" ratio.

The standard dependency ratio is usually defined as the ratio of the economically dependent population to the population in the age group that can be expected to support itself and others economically through work. The latter group is generally defined as those aged 15–64 years, whereas those under the age of 15 or over 64 are considered dependent because they are either too young or too old to be expected to support themselves. A high dependency ratio suggests there is greater stress placed on those aged 15–64 as they must then support more "others" in addition to supporting themselves.

The standard dependency ratio considers only financial dependency. For the UNRISD project, the care dependency ratio is intended to reflect the relative burden placed on carers in society. As with the standard ratio, the care dependency ratio is defined in terms of age groups. This is likely to undercount the number needing care, as it does not take into consideration those in the carer age group who are disabled or ill to the extent that they need care. The undercount is probably most marked in respect of South Africa and Tanzania, where the AIDS epidemic has significantly increased the likelihood that an adult will need care. It was, however, not possible to include this factor in the ratio because, for Tanzania, reliable data on HIV prevalence and data distinguishing the AIDS sick from those who are HIV positive were not available. The ratio also disregards the fact that all people need a certain amount of care. The ratio was nevertheless considered useful in allowing comparisons between the relative burden across countries and across time.[1]

To provide some nuance, the ratio distinguishes between those needing intensive care and those needing a lesser level of care. The former include those aged 0–6 years and those aged 85 years and older, and are given a full weight. The latter are those aged 7–12 years and 75–84 years, and are given a weight of 0.5.[2] The potential carers are defined as those aged 15–74 years, all of whom are given a full weight. Those aged 13 or 14 years are not included in the calculation on the assumption that they will be able to provide more or less the same amount of care as they receive. Their inclusion in both the nominator and denominator would change some of the ratios, but the likely effect was not considered big enough to warrant including them on both sides of the "care equation".

The calculation can thus be summarised as follows:

Those needing care in all countries:

A = 0–6 years; weight: 1
B = 7–12 years; weight: 0.5
C = 75–84 years; weight: 0.5
D = 85+; weight: 1

Potential care givers in all countries:

E = 15–74 years

Care dependency ratio = (A+B+C+D)/E

Figure 1.8 shows the resultant care ratios. The ratio is lowest for Japan and the Republic of Korea, and highest for Nicaragua. The ranking to some

What do Time Use Studies Tell Us about Unpaid Care Work? 33

extent matches the relative fertility rates, with a higher ratio in countries with higher total fertility rate. This match is, however, far from exact. For example, Tanzania and Nicaragua have very similar care dependency ratios, but the total fertility rate for Nicaragua was around 3.0 in the period 2000–2005, while that for Tanzania was 5.7 (UNDP 2007:243ff). This particular anomaly might be partly explained by the severity of the HIV/AIDS epidemic in Tanzania, and the fact that it tends to increase the infant mortality rate.

The differences in the actual levels are large—ranging from 0.18 to 0.61. This suggests that a caregiver in the Republic of Korea would, on average, share the responsibility for caring for a single person with at least five other people, while a caregiver in Nicaragua or Tanzania would be responsible for more than half of all the care needed by another person.

In order to understand how such large differences arise, Figure 1.9 illustrates the components that make up the care dependency ratio. The components are reflected as weighted. The figure suggests that the size of the population aged 0–6 years is a major determinant of the care dependency ratio, followed by the population aged 7–14 years. (The ratio for Tanzania may be slightly exaggerated by clustering of the sample at age 4. This could have been caused by fieldworkers wanting to avoid having to ask all the child labour–related questions of this group.) While the older age groups are most evident in the Japan and city of Buenos Aires samples, they account for much less of a care-giving burden than the children. (The care dependency ratio for Argentina as a whole is somewhat higher, at 0.21.)

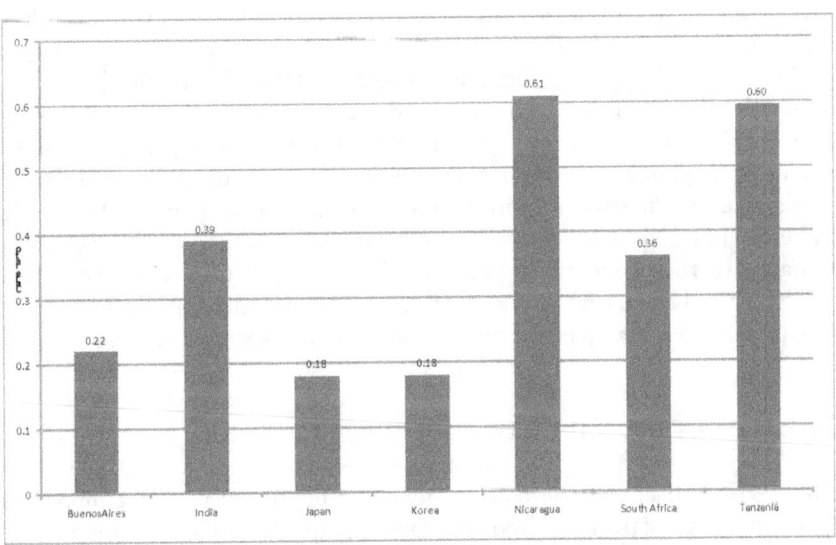

Figure 1.8 Care dependency ratios.

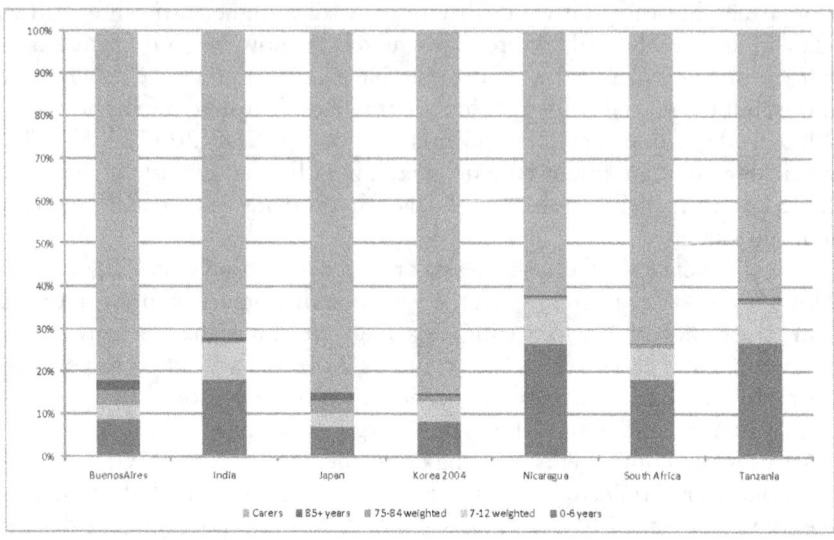

Figure 1.9 Components of care dependency ratios.

Comparison of the care dependency ratios, with the amount of time spent on care of persons as shown in Figure 1.6, suggests that, contrary to expectation, the amount of time spent on care of persons tends to be larger where care dependency ratios are low, and vice versa. Thus the city of Buenos Aires has one of the lowest care dependency ratios, but the mean time spent by women aged 15–64 years on care of persons is higher than for all other countries. Conversely, Tanzania has the second highest care dependency ratio, even before considering the HIV–related need for care, although women in this country record less time spent on care of persons than in all other countries. This counter-intuitive finding might to some extent be explained by the fact that where families have many children, someone can take care of more than one child simultaneously. One would therefore not expect the amount of time spent on care to increase proportionately to the proportion of children in the population. However, there are clearly other factors at play that also determine the time people in different countries perceive and report themselves as spending on care.

THE MONETARY VALUE OF UNPAID CARE WORK

This section discusses the country teams' attempts to assign a monetary value to unpaid care work and compares the resultant values with a range of macroeconomic measures. This exercise is in accordance with the SNA recommendation that, although unpaid care work should not (currently) be included in the calculation of GDP, countries should compile "satellite accounts" that reflect this work and its value to the economy.

Undertaking this valuation is not intended to imply that this work should necessarily be paid. It is also not meant to imply that money could accurately reflect the real value of the work for society. Instead its purpose is to promote more "accurate and comprehensive" valuation of the work that takes place in economies (UNDP 1995:98), and to provide support for arguments that those who do this work are entitled to a fair share of, and control over, the income generated by the paid work done by members of their family or household.

As will be discussed in the following section, there are many complications associated with the exercise. There are, however, also far more complications and heroic assumptions associated with the estimation of GDP than most who use this measure generally recognise. Despite the complications, a measure on unpaid care work that reflects pesos, rupees, rand, shillings, yen or won, might have greater success in attracting the attention of economists than measures that simply record time. Assigning monetary value to care also allows comparison with a range of other macroeconomic measures, thus highlighting the relative importance of care in the different economies.

Deriving the Value of Unpaid Care Work

The underlying idea behind assigning a monetary value to unpaid care work is to estimate the number of hours worked, and multiply this by some measure of hourly earnings. As described in more detail in Budlender and Brathaug (2002), there are four basic standard approaches to choosing the measure of hourly earnings, namely:

- the average earnings approach;
- the opportunity cost approach;
- the generalist approach; and
- the specialist approach.

The first two approaches have as an underlying question: how much would a person undertaking unpaid care work have earned in the market if the person had performed paid work rather than unpaid care work? The first approach uses the average earnings for all people (or all people of a particular sex) in the economy, while the second approach uses the actual earnings of the person who did the unpaid care work. Because of the underlying question (what would the person earn in the labour market?) and because average female earnings are usually markedly lower than male ones, even where they have equal educational qualifications, the first approach is usually sex-disaggregated. This tends to result in a lower overall estimate of the value of unpaid care work because the greater number of hours worked by women is multiplied by a lower value, lowering the overall estimate. Wolf (2004:117) notes that some researchers reject this approach because it reflects the gender discrimination in the labour market. However, if one accepts the underlying question as being what a person would otherwise have earned doing paid work, then existing discrimination must be reflected if a realistic estimate is to be arrived at. Disaggregation does not imply endorsement of the lower earnings that women earn in paid work. Instead, it reflects the fact that female actors would be likely to earn less than male actors if they substituted paid work for the unpaid care work.

The next two approaches have the following underlying question: how much would a household need to pay someone else to do the unpaid care work, that is, the replacement cost? As Wolf (2004:118) argues, this estimate reflects the savings achieved by not paying for this work on the market.

The generalist approach uses the average wage paid to a worker, such as a domestic worker or housekeeper, who would carry out virtually all the tasks. The specialist approach assumes that the household employs a specialist to do each of the different types of work. For example, the household would employ a cook or chef to prepare meals, a nursemaid or teacher to perform various tasks associated with childcare, a nurse to care for ill people, and so on. For this approach, the calculations are not sex-disaggregated as, in theory the household's concern would be to have the work performed rather than with the gender of the worker. In practice, for the domestic worker approach, the overwhelming majority of workers in most countries are female.

The UNRISD project used two approaches—the average earnings approach and the generalist approach. The opportunity cost approach was not pursued because of its theoretical and practical limitations. On the theoretical side, for example, this approach assumes that a meal prepared by a university professor has more value than one prepared by an unskilled worker, even if the same ingredients are used. On the practical side, there are difficulties in assigning a value to the time of someone who is not employed. The specialist approach was avoided because of its complexity, and because of the difficulty of finding appropriate paid workers for all tasks. Both these choices do, however, tend to result in lower estimates of the value of unpaid care work.

For both the average earnings and generalist approaches, two variants were possible. For average earnings, the first, and preferred, variant was based on the average earnings of all employed people with non-zero earnings, whether they were employees or self-employed. The second variant, using only employee wages, was the only possible option for Japan and India, given the non-availability of reliable information on self-employed earnings. For India, the available wage data are for regular salaries or waged employees in farm and non-farm enterprises, and spanning both organised and unorganised, including domestic workers. The non-availability of self-employed earnings is, however, unfortunate as the self-employed account for about half of all employed people in India, and their earnings are generally lower than those of regular employees, with much of the work unpaid. The second variant was also calculated for several countries, even where earnings more generally were available. For the city of Buenos Aires and the Republic of Korea, where the informal sector is not significant, there is little difference in the value of the average earnings and average wage variants.

For the generalist approach, the first variant entailed the inclusion of all occupations involving work similar to housework, such as cleaning and cooking, whether performed in institutions or in the home. Technically, this generally included a range of occupations in major category 5 of the International Standard Classification of Occupations or its equivalent. Teachers were excluded in the measures reported in the following, except in the case of Argentina. Although some teaching includes a large measure of care, teachers were excluded because they constituted a relatively large presence in most countries, and their wages—which are generally higher than those of the average domestic worker, cleaner or cook—would have skewed the value upward. The second variant focused only on wages of domestic workers more narrowly defined. Nicaragua included the reported value of in-kind earnings for this variant. In Argentina the hourly wage for domestic workers was found to be similar to that for other social services, excluding education. The research report (Esquivel 2008) notes, however, that actual earnings of domestic workers tend to be lower than those of the other workers because hours worked are likely to be fewer, and there are usually no added benefits.

In almost all cases the earnings data were sourced from household surveys. It is well-known that respondents tend to under-report earnings in such surveys. No correction was made for this, as the extent of the under-reporting is not reliably known either for the employed population as a whole, or in terms of its variation across groups. This lack of correction for under-reporting usually results in lower estimates of the value of unpaid care work.

Further downward bias results from the fact that all approaches to valuation reflect gender discrimination in the labour market. Thus the opportunity cost/average earnings approach is biased downward because women tend to do more care work than men and also to have lower earnings. The replacement cost approach is biased downward because it uses earnings of care workers, who are predominantly women, and tend to have lower earnings than many others in the economy.

In all countries, only non-zero earnings were considered when calculating the various averages and means. This choice inflates the value for countries such as Tanzania and India, where large numbers of employed people work unpaid on family farms or in family businesses. In Tanzania, for example, 64 per cent of employed people were reported to be working on their own farm or *shamba* in 2006, with a further 16 per cent doing unpaid work in family businesses or agriculture. Similarly, when calculating the first variant of the generalist wage for Tanzania, only 16 per cent of the relevant respondents were found to record non-zero wages.

A choice, which again results in lower estimates for some countries, is the use of median earnings rather than mean earnings for the averages. There are two reasons for this choice, one theoretical and one practical. Theoretically, the median is chosen because earnings tend to be clustered at the lower end. The mean thus tends to over-state the true "middle". Practically, using the median avoids the problem of how to deal with outliers in the data, at least some of which probably represent incorrect capture of data. The results presented in the following section for Nicaragua, South Africa and Tanzania are based on values using medians rather than means. For Argentina, the median is used for all but the generalist approach.

Each country team was free to choose what age group to include when valuing unpaid care work. India and Nicaragua focused on the age group 15–64 years, even though their data covered a larger age group. Other countries used the age group covered in their time use survey.

All countries valued at least two aggregates of unpaid care work, the first relating to unpaid care work as a whole and the second relating to care of persons. For unpaid care work, the scope was very similar across countries, except that Nicaragua, South Africa and Tanzania included the collection of fuel and water. This was done because the primary comparison was with GDP, and the collection of fuel and water is not included when calculating GDP in these countries (and most others). In any event, for Argentina, Japan and the Republic of Korea, this activity would not have been significant.

There was more variation in what was included in the care of persons aggregate. Nicaragua used only unpaid care of children. All other countries included care of persons in the respondent's household. Argentina, South Africa and Tanzania also included care of adults and children in other households.

Comparisons with Macroeconomic Indicators

The first comparison is with GDP. This comparison is important as the basis for advocacy that aims to change the SNA rules so that the production boundary includes unpaid production of services for one's own use, just as they were changed in 1993—as a result of advocacy—to cover subsistence production of goods and the collection of fuel and water. Essentially, the GDP comparisons provide support for the argument that the amount of unpaid care work done and its value are too large to be ignored in economic decision-making.

Figure 1.10 shows the results of the comparison with GDP in respect of both unpaid care work (left) and care of persons (right). (For Argentina, the value of unpaid care work was compared with the gross geographical product for the city of Buenos Aires.) The value of unpaid care work is estimated to be between 7 per cent (using the generalist wage in Argentina) and 63 per cent (using the employee wage in India and earnings in Tanzania) of GDP. For care of persons, the range is between 1 per cent (using the domestic worker wage in South Africa) and 14 per cent (using employee wages in India). The high measures for India and Tanzania could be regarded as misleading to the extent that many workers doing GDP/SNA work in these countries are unpaid, and GDP is thus probably lower than it would otherwise be.

The figure shows substantial variation in the percentage for each of the two values, both between and within countries using different measures. The variation in values within country is particularly marked in the case of India and South Africa. In both these countries the highest value for unpaid care work (or person care) is more than twice as high as the lowest value. One reason for this is the very low wages paid to domestic workers in both these countries when compared to wages of other employees. In South Africa, for example, the median wage recorded for domestic workers is R2.60 per hour compared to R7.75 per hour for all employees. In the Republic of Korea, in contrast, the domestic worker wage measure is higher than the generalist measure. Nevertheless, across all countries the generalist and domestic worker measures are lower than the average earnings and average wage measures. This is, in part, a reflection of the dominance of females in care-related occupations and the relatively low wages paid for these types of work. For the countries where there is a measure in respect of both average earnings and average wages, the measures tend to be very

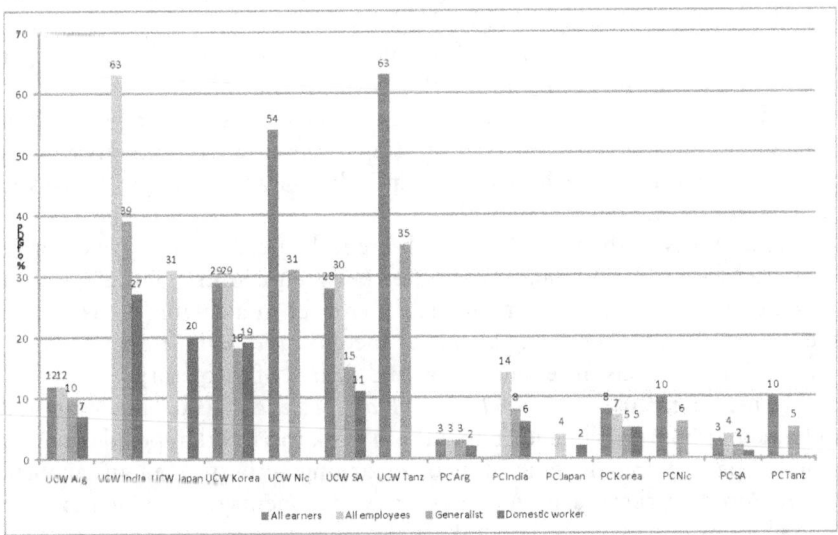

Figure 1.10 Value of unpaid care work and care of persons as a precentage of GDP.

similar. The biggest difference in this respect is found for South Africa, which has a bigger informal sector than the other two countries—Argentina and the Republic of Korea—which have both measures.

Comparison of the GDP-related patterns with those reflecting "volume" of unpaid care work and SNA work shown in Figure 1.4 illustrates the extent to which differences in the earnings used for valuation affect the value attributed to unpaid care work. For example, while South Africa has among the lowest values for unpaid care work in the GDP comparison, the volume analysis suggests that it is higher than for all other countries except Nicaragua.

Comparisons were also made with a few further macroeconomic measures. To simplify presentation, the following graphs show the results only in respect of unpaid care work.

The first comparison is with the *value of paid work* in the economy. This comparison is an alternative version of the volume comparison presented in Figure 1.4. The two main differences with the volume comparison are, first, that the hours of paid and unpaid work performed are multiplied by relevant earnings and, second, unpaid SNA work is excluded.

The value for paid work used in the comparison was generally obtained from the same survey as the time use data or another household survey. For Argentina, Nicaragua, South Africa and Tanzania, the value represents the income of all earners, whether employees or self-employed. For India, the value represents income of regular salaried employees. Similarly, in Japan and the Republic of Korea only employees are included in the calculation. This restriction will have more of an impact on the Indian comparison than the Japan or Korean comparisons, given the high levels of self-employment in India.

Figure 1.11 shows the value of unpaid care work ranging from 19 per cent (domestic worker wage in South Africa) of the value of paid work in the economy to 190 per cent (all earners in Nicaragua). The high value in Nicaragua could be regarded as misleading to the extent that it only reflects SNA work that is paid. The low value in India is interesting, given that the comparison is only with employees.

The patterns in the preceding graph are influenced by the type of earnings used for the valuation. These differ between countries for a range of reasons, including different methods, differences in available datasets and the degree of under-reporting of earned income, and real differences in the economies, the levels of remuneration and degree of inequality.

The next comparison is with *personal tax revenue*. Ingrid Palmer (quoted in Bakker 1993:6) has likened unpaid care work to a tax that people (mainly women) pay before engaging in income-earning activity. Men and women are required, if they earn enough, to pay a monetary tax which is their contribution to the public good. This tax is more often paid by men, and men tend to pay more of this tax than women. Most women and some men, irrespective of whether they earn, also contribute through their unpaid care

What do Time Use Studies Tell Us about Unpaid Care Work? 41

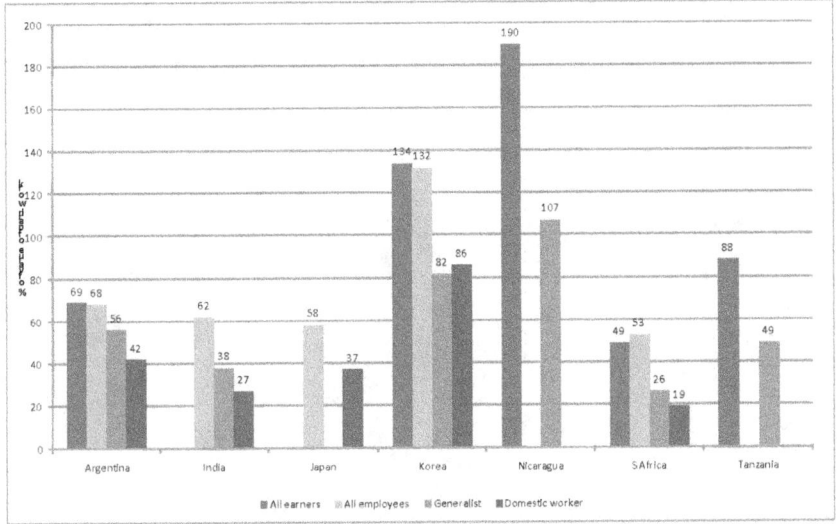

Figure 1.11 Value of unpaid care work as a precentage of paid work in the economy.

work to the public good. Indeed, in 2001, Germany's highest court ruled that it was unconstitutional to tax parents at the same rate as the childless, given that parents "produce the future workers needed to keep the system solvent" (Wolf 2004:126–127).

The unpaid care work "tax" contribution can constrain the carers' opportunities to earn monetary income. Further, the unpaid care tax adds a regressive element to the tax system given that, overall, women (who do most of the care) tend to be poorer in monetary terms than men. The regressive element is increased to the extent that, in some countries at least, poorer people tend to do more unpaid care work than wealthier ones. It is therefore interesting to compare the value of unpaid care work with various tax measures.

Figure 1.12 compares the value of unpaid care work with measures of *personal tax*. For India and Japan the comparison is with personal tax revenue, for Nicaragua with income tax revenue, for South Africa with personal and individual tax revenue, and for Tanzania with individual income tax revenue. In the Republic of Korea, the comparison is with the total for direct taxes, which include income, corporation, inheritance and gift, and comprehensive real estate holding taxes.

In this graph, the low values for the Republic of Korea and South Africa are explained by the fact that both countries have substantial formal sectors with relatively effective taxation of those employed in these sectors. The higher values for Japan are therefore noteworthy as one would expect a similarly substantial formal sector and effective taxation in this country.

42 *Debbie Budlender*

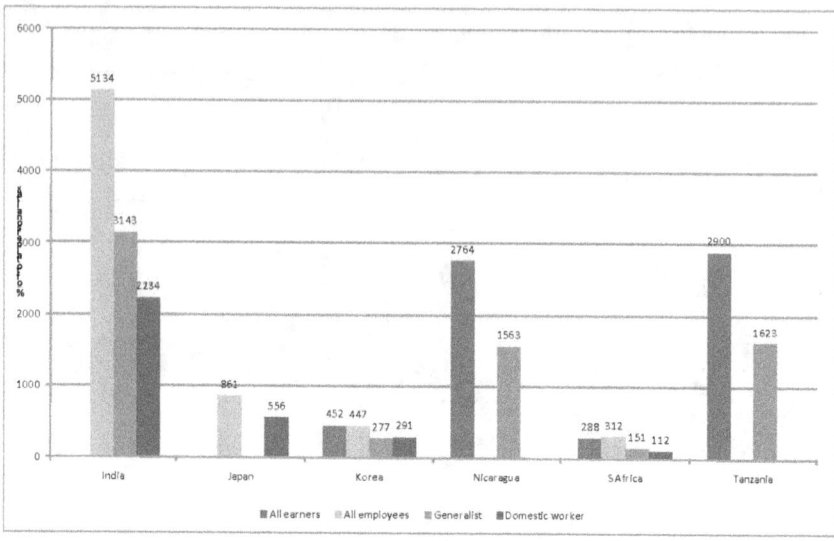

Figure 1.12 Value of unpaid care work as precentage of personal tax.

The other countries, with large proportions of the population engaged in informal and unregistered work, show much larger percentages when comparing unpaid care work and personal tax. For India, in particular, the highest measure shows unpaid care work equivalent to 5,134 per cent of the value of personal tax revenue.

The preceding comparisons show very different patterns for the different countries, and variation across the different comparisons. The variation is the result of differences in the labour market, including the level of inequality in earnings by gender and occupation; and differences in the distribution of care provision across the home, market and state. Unpaid care work tends to loom larger, in comparative terms, in less developed countries because of the smaller size of government and the paid economy. It is consistently less than one might otherwise expect in South Africa because of the extreme inequalities in earnings, which result in particularly low (relative) earnings for care work and for women, which in turn influenced the value ascribed to unpaid care work. Nevertheless, across all countries, the relative size of unpaid care work is sufficiently large that it is difficult to justify ignoring it in policy-making.

CONCLUSION

This chapter has shown some constant basic gender patterns in engagement in SNA and unpaid care work across seven countries: Argentina, India, Japan, the Republic of Korea, Nicaragua, South Africa and Tanzania. As expected, men are more likely than women to engage in SNA work, and to do so for longer than women, while women are more likely than men to engage in unpaid care work and care of persons, and to do so for longer than men. The analysis has also confirmed that across countries a range of similar factors influences the amount of time spent on unpaid care work and care of persons: work (employment) status, having children in the household, being married and age. Other factors that reflect social standing—such as income, caste, race and educational achievement—also influence participation in, and the amount of time spent on care. Here, however, the patterns vary to some extent across countries.

Overall, there are at least as many differences as similarities. In particular, there are significant variations in the "size" of care work undertaken in the sense of the level of participation rates, average times spent by women and men on different activities, and absolute and relative differences between women and men. Some of these variations reflect methodological differences in terms of instruments, number of days covered, classification schemes, age group covered, and so on. However, the methodological differences cannot explain away more than a small proportion of the differences.

This finding of diversity should not be surprising. Nor should the difficulty of finding simple reasons for some of the patterns be a cause for surprise. In this respect, Pacholok and Gauthier's (2004) examination of patterns in respect of paid work, housework and childcare in Canada, Germany, Italy and Sweden confirms that in developed countries, too, even quite simple hypotheses are not supported in any simple way by the available data.

Pacholok and Gauthier test four hypotheses:

- countries with a smaller wage gap between women and men will exhibit a less marked division of labour;
- the extent to which a country's population has traditional beliefs in respect of gender will increase the gender gaps;
- the existence of opportunities for reducing the time spent in paid work, for example, through availability of part-time work, will result in more time being spent with children; and
- the level of state support for families will increase the time spent with children.

These hypotheses are interesting in that they touch on issues, such as the influence of government policies and practices, that were a core focus of analysis within the UNRISD project on *Political and Social Economy of Care*. However, despite restricting the analysis to dual-earner couples so as to avoid confounding factors, it is only for the third of these hypotheses that Pacholok and Gauthier find real support. Even then the support is "partial" (Pacholok and Gauthier 2004:215–216). Clearly, the determinants of the types and amounts of work done by women and men are complicated. With the much more diverse set of countries used in the UNRISD project, and without the restriction to dual-earner couples, the variation is not all that surprising.

Essentially time use surveys offer a way to measure the gender division of labour, which many consider to be an underlying feature of gender patterns and inequality in society. The differences found between countries in this chapter serve to confirm that gender is not "god-given" and immutable. Instead, it is something that varies across countries and cultures.

For policy purposes, however, what happens in a particular country is as important, if not more so, than cross-country comparisons. This chapter and the country chapters present cross-sectional comparisons of different groups within a particular country at a particular point in time. Also needed are longitudinal comparisons of patterns of time use within the same country. Of the countries covered in this book, longitudinal data are available only for Japan and Korea, and the chapters on these countries present some analysis of trends.

All countries need to conduct time use surveys at regular intervals, using a standard methodology that allows reliable comparisons over time, similar to the current practice of ongoing labour force surveys. However, time use surveys would not need to be conducted as regularly as some countries conduct labour force surveys because time use patterns are unlikely to shift as quickly, unless there are economic shocks, major disasters and epidemics or policy shifts in areas such as public support for childcare.

NOTES

1. After calculating this ratio, the research team discovered that a similar index, named the Madrid Scale, was used in a publication on gender equality in Latin America and the Caribbean (Montaño 2007). While the age groups used differ somewhat between the Madrid Scale and the UNRISD approach, the two measures are very similar.
2. In Argentina and Japan the presence of a child under 6 years of age was used, while in South Africa and Tanzania it was a child under 7 years of age; in the Republic of Korea the cut-off age was 8 years old, and in India and Nicaragua it was 18 years old.

REFERENCES

Bakker, Isabella. 1993. *Engendering Macroeconomic Analysis: Conceptual Silences and New Research Strategies.* Paper prepared for the International Studies Association Meetings, 23–27 March, Acapulco.
Bittman, Michael. 2004. "Parenthood without penalty: Time-use and public policy in Australia and Finland." In N. Folbre and M. Bittman (eds.), *Family Time: The Social Organization of Care.* Routledge, London.

Bittman, Michael, Lyn Craig and Nancy Folbre. 2004. "Packaging care: What happens when children receive non-parental care?" In N. Folbre and M. Bittman (eds.), *Family Time: The Social Organization of Care*. Routledge, London.

Bittman, Michael and Judy Wajcman. 2004. "The rush hour: The quality of leisure time and gender equity." In N. Folbre and M. Bittman (eds.), *Family Time: The Social Organization of Care*. Routledge, London.

Budig, Michelle J. and Nancy Folbre. 2004. "Activity, proximity, or responsibility: Measuring parental childcare time." in N. Folbre and M. Bittman (eds.), *Family Time: The Social Organization of Care*. Routledge, London.

Budlender, Debbie. 2007. *A Critical Review of Selected Time Use Surveys*. Programme on Gender and Development, Paper No. 2. UNRISD, Geneva.

Budlender, Debbie and Ann Lisbet Brathaug. 2002. *Calculating the Value of Unpaid Labour: A Discussion Document*. Statistics South Africa, Pretoria.

Elson D. 2000. *Progress of the World's Women 2000: UNIFEM Biennial Report*. United Nations Development Fund for Women, New York.

Esquivel, Valeria. 2008. *Political and Social Economy of Care: Research Report 2 on Argentina*. UNRISD, Geneva.

Franzoni, Juliana Martinez. 2005 "La pieza que faltaba: Uso del tiempo y regímenes de bienestar en América Latina." *Nueva Soicedad*, Vol. 199, pp. 35–52, September-October.

Hoffmann, E. and A. Mata. 1998. "Measuring working time: An alternative approach to classifying time use." *Bulletin of Labour Statistics*, No. 3.

Ironmonger, Duncan. 2004. "Bringing up Bobby and Betty: The inputs and outputs of childcare time." In N. Folbre and M. Bittman (eds.), *Family Time: The Social Organization of Care*. Routledge, London.

Jelin, Elizabeth (ed.). 1990. *Women and Social Change in Latin America*. UNRISD and Zed Books, London.

Meena, Ruth. 2007. *Political and Social Economy of Care: Research Report 1 on Tanzania*. UNRISD, Geneva.

Montaño S. 2007. *El aporte de las mujeres a la igualdad en América Latina y el Caribe*. Conferencia Regional Sobre La Mujer de América Latina y el Caribe. Unidad Mujer ye Desarrollo de la CEPAL, Santiago de Chile.

Pacholok, Shelley and Anne H. Gauthier. 2004. "A tale of dual-earner families in four countries." In N. Folbre and M. Bittman (eds.), *Family Time: The Social Organization of Care*. Routledge, London.

Razavi, S. 2007. *The Political and Social Economy of Care in a Development Context: Contextual Issues, Research Questions, and Policy Options*. Programme on Gender and Development, Paper No. 3. UNRISD, Geneva.

Smeeding, Timothy M. and Joseph T. Marchand. 2004. "Family time and public policy in the United States." In N. Folbre and M. Bittman (eds.), *Family Time: The Social Organization of Care*. Routledge, London.

United Nations. 1996. *The World's Women 1995: Trends and Statistics*. Department for Economic and Social Information and Policy Analysis. United Nations: New York.

United Nations Development Programme (UNDP). 2007. *Human Development Report 2007/2008: Fighting Climate Change: Human Solidarity in a Divided World*. Oxford University Press, New York.

United Nations Development Programme. 1995. *Human Development Report 2005*. Oxford University Press, New York.

Wolf, Douglas A. 2004. "Valuing informal elder care." In N. Folbre and M. Bittman (eds.), *Family Time: The Social Organization of Care*. Routledge, London.

2 Tanzania
Care in the Context of HIV and AIDS
Debbie Budlender

INTRODUCTION

This chapter explores the data from the time use module of the Tanzanian Integrated Labour Force Survey (ILFS) carried out by the National Bureau of Statistics in 2006. The 2006 time use module of the ILFS represented the first time that the National Bureau of Statistics had attempted this type of investigation. Every fifth household sampled for the ILFS was included in the sample for the time use module. The realised sample for the survey was over 3,000 households. All members of the household aged 5 years and older were targeted, yielding a realised sample of 10,553 respondents with valid diary information after cleaning. The data were weighted so as to be representative of the country's population aged 5 years and older as a whole. At the time the ILFS was conducted, the country's population aged 5 years and older was estimated at close to 30 million people.

Each targeted household member was meant to be visited for seven consecutive days, and asked what they had done during each hour of the previous day. For each hourly "slot", respondents could name up to five activities. The relatively long period of 1 hour was used because the designers felt that respondents, many of whom would be rural, less educated people, would not be able to report activities in terms of shorter time-slots. Where more than one activity was reported for a particular slot, the respondent was required to specify whether each activity was done simultaneously or separately from other activities

The Tanzanian time use module utilised a slightly adapted version of the United Nations' trial classification for time use surveys. Table 2.1 shows the distribution of time spent per day by the average male and female aged 5 years and older according to the ten basic categories. The first three of these represent SNA work, the following three represent unpaid care work, and the remaining four represent non-productive activities.

In reality, there are 1,440 minutes in a day, and the minutes columns should reflect this as the total as the 24-hour minute measure was used for this tabulation. Table 2.1 was, however, generated using an early version of the data which had not been fully cleaned, hence the totals of 1,451 minutes for males and 1,448 minutes for females. This should, however, not affect the overall patterns. The table already reveals that a relatively small proportion of the day is spent on care for household members, but that females tend to spend nearly three times as long as males on this activity. This and other patterns are explored in more detail in subsequent sections. The table also reveals that, as in other countries, a large proportion of time is spent on personal care (of self) and self-maintenance, a category that covers activities such as sleeping, eating and dressing.

DESCRIPTION OF THE SURVEY POPULATION

A standard set of disaggregations were used to explore patterns in time use among different groups, namely by age group, marital status, presence of children under 7 years of age in the household, employment status, educational achievement, geographical area (rural/urban), household income

Table 2.1 Distribution of Time Spent on Activities Per Day by Sex

	Male		Female	
	Minutes	%	Minutes	%
Employment for establishments	90	6%	35	2%
Primary production activities	181	12%	164	11%
Non-primary, non-establishment productions	6	0%	7	0%
Household maintenance etc.	53	4%	170	12%
Care of children, the sick, elderly, disabled	12	1%	35	2%
Community services and help to other hhs	9	1%	7	0%
Learning	88	6%	76	5%
Social and cultural activities	131	9%	96	7%
Mass media use	18	1%	8	1%
Personal care and self-maintenance	863	60%	850	59%
Total	1451	100%	1448	100%

level, and household composition. All of these were cross-tabulated by sex, given the importance of gender in shaping time use.

Three age groups are used, representing children (5–17 years), the primary reproductive and productive years (18–49 years) and the ones in which having young children is most likely, and those who are older (50 years and older). For the purposes of this chapter, these groups are referred to as children, adults and older people. The middle group accounts for close on half of the weighted sample, with the children accounting for nearly two-fifths. The age distribution across male and female is fairly similar, but with more women in the older age groups. This reflects greater female longevity. In much of the following analysis we focus only on those aged 18 years and older so as to remove the confounding effects of combining children and adults.

Almost half of the total sample population is "single" in the sense of never having been married or lived together with a partner, but this percentage drops to 19 per cent when analysis is restricted to adults. The married group accounts for 42 per cent of the total sample, and two-thirds (66 per cent) of adults. Males are noticeably less likely than females to be recorded as widowed or divorced. The gender pattern in respect of widowed people reflects the different age compositions as well as the tendency for women to marry men older than themselves. The widowed and divorced groups are too small for reliable analysis in respect of males.

Analysis in respect of co-residence with children differentiates between those who live in a household that has no children younger than 7 years and those in households with at least one child under this age. This differentiation is made on the basis that children under seven tend to need more care than older children, and are also less likely than older children to spend part of their day in school. The children concerned need not necessarily be the biological offspring of the respondent.

Over two-thirds of all respondents live in households with young children, and when analysis is restricted to adults, the percentage falls slightly, to 63 per cent. Women are slightly more likely than men to be living in households with young children.

Analysis of work status utilises the standard labour force categories of employed (i.e. having done SNA-type work in the last calendar week), unemployed (i.e. not having done SNA-type work, but having been available for work), and not economically active (NEA i.e. not having done SNA-type work). The categorisation is based on the standard international definition of employment. What is unusual in Tanzania, but nevertheless in line with international recommendations, is that the category of employed includes those whose only SNA work was collection of fuel and water. This group accounts for a very small proportion of the employed because most adults are also engaged in some other form of employment. Most of those whose only economic activity is collection of fuel and water are adult women living in Dar es Salaam, as adult women in this city are less likely than other women to be doing other forms of economic work. Thus collection of fuel and water accounts for a full 35 per cent of secondary activities among women, but these women would usually have another main economic activity. The inclusion of collection of fuel and water when defining employment should not skew the findings in any noticeable way because of the small proportion recording this as their main activity.

The overwhelming majority of adult men (93 per cent) and adult women (87 per cent) are recorded as employed, with the percentages at 73 per cent and 68 per cent respectively when children are included. Unemployed people account for a very small proportion of the population and disaggregation for this group is unlikely to be reliable. The NEA group is substantial for the full sample where it includes children who are not working because of schooling, but constitutes only 6 per cent of the adult sample.

More than a quarter of respondents are recorded as never having attended formal schooling, with less than 1 per cent having tertiary education. The biggest single grouping consists of those with primary schooling, who account for around two-thirds of respondents. The tertiary group is clearly too small for separate analysis and is combined with the secondary group, which is also relatively small, in the following analysis. A small number, virtually all children, are recorded as having no education. This group is combined with the "never attended" group in further analysis and labelled as "none". There are marked gender patterns, which become stronger when children are excluded, in that 35 per cent of adult women but "only" 21 per cent of adult men have never attended formal schooling. Conversely, the percentage of adult women with secondary education or above is only 6 per cent, compared to 10 per cent for adult men.

Three-quarters of the full sample is recorded in rural areas, with a slightly lower percentage of adults recorded in rural areas. The patterns for male and female are very similar.

The time use questionnaire asks about household income using income categories. More than half of respondents live in households with average incomes below Tshs. 50,000 per month, the lowest pre-specified category. A further 28 per cent of respondents live in households with monthly incomes between Tshs. 50,000 and Tshs. 99,000. The patterns for the sample as a whole and for adults only are very similar. Among adults, males are perhaps slightly more likely than females to live in wealthier households.

The final form of disaggregation investigated is based on household composition. To arrive at the different categories, we use combinations of the same three age groups as before. For example, if a household contains at least one member from each of the categories, it is "Ch+Ad+Old" (Child, adult and older person), whereas if it has no member in the adult category but at least one member in each of the other categories, it is "Ch+Old". These three categories between them yield seven possible different combinations. The number of respondents reporting that they live in a household consisting only of children is, however, so small (less than 1 per cent) that it is not worth reporting on. The "adult and older" and "old" categories are also omitted from further analysis as they are too small to produce reliable results.

Among the remaining households, those with children and adults are most common, followed by those consisting of all three "generations". Women are somewhat more likely than men to be members of all the household combinations which include children, with one or more percentage points between the female and male percentages in this category for all three household groupings containing children. In contrast, adult-only households are more common for men than women.

PAID AND UNPAID WORK

The first set of time use tabulations focuses on the amount of time spent by individuals from different groups on what is often loosely referred to as paid and unpaid work. To tighten the analysis, and to illustrate the differences resulting from different conceptions, the tables show patterns in respect of two measures of what might loosely be termed "paid work" and two measures of what might loosely be termed "unpaid work".

There are three categories in the activity classification system used in Tanzania that together cover SNA work, namely (a) employment for establishments; (b) primary production activities not for establishments; and (c) services for income and other production of goods not for establishments. The following analysis uses all three of these categories as a broad measure of "paid work", and the first and third categories as a narrow measure. The measures are not exact because, for example, the first and third categories would include unpaid non-agricultural SNA work for establishments or non-establishments respectively, or unpaid help in a family business. The second category includes a large amount of work that is unpaid. In particular, it includes substantial subsistence work in agriculture and collection of fuel and water. The SNA category also includes time reported as being spent seeking employment.

The categories making up unpaid care work are (a) household maintenance, management and shopping for own household; (b) care for children, the sick, elderly and disabled for own household; and (c) community services and help to other households. For the broad measure of unpaid work below all three categories are used. For the narrow measure, termed "care of persons", only (b) is used. Again, these measures are not exact. For example, (c) includes several care of persons activities that relate to non-household members. Nevertheless, the following analysis should give a good idea of the balance (or lack of it) between paid and unpaid work for different groups.

This set of tabulations focuses on the average time spent per day by all members of a group on particular categories of activity, with the average calculated over all members, whether or not they engaged in that activity. Later analysis will investigate the extent of involvement of members of particular groups by looking at the number of "actors". The tabulations use the 24-hour minute. Because the Tanzanian time use module collected seven days' activities for most respondents, the reported time spent on each activity by a particular person was divided by the number of days for which they reported activities.

The 24-hour minute undercounts activities which are done simultaneously in that the available time is then divided equally between the simultaneous activities. Later analysis in this chapter uses a "full-hour" minute which drops the 24-hour limitation and measures full duration. Unpaid care work activities—and personal care in particular—is more likely than SNA work activities to be reported as having been done simultaneously. Thus the ratio of "full minutes" to 24-hour minutes is 1.00 or 1.01 for two of the three SNA categories, while it is 1.07 for household care. Household care has the highest ratio of all of the ten categories except media use, where the ratio is a high 1.18.

Figure 2.1 uses a simple male/female split for the population aged 5 years and older to illustrate how two of the reported categories form subsets of the other two reported categories. Thus the males in the sample spend, on average, 19 per cent of their day on SNA work, which is made up of 7 per cent of the day on "paid work" as defined, and a further 12 per cent on subsistence-type work. In contrast, females spend 14 per cent of their day on SNA work, which is made up of 3 per cent on "paid work" and 11 per cent on subsistence-type work. In respect of unpaid work, males spent a total of 5 per cent on unpaid care work, compared to 14 per cent for

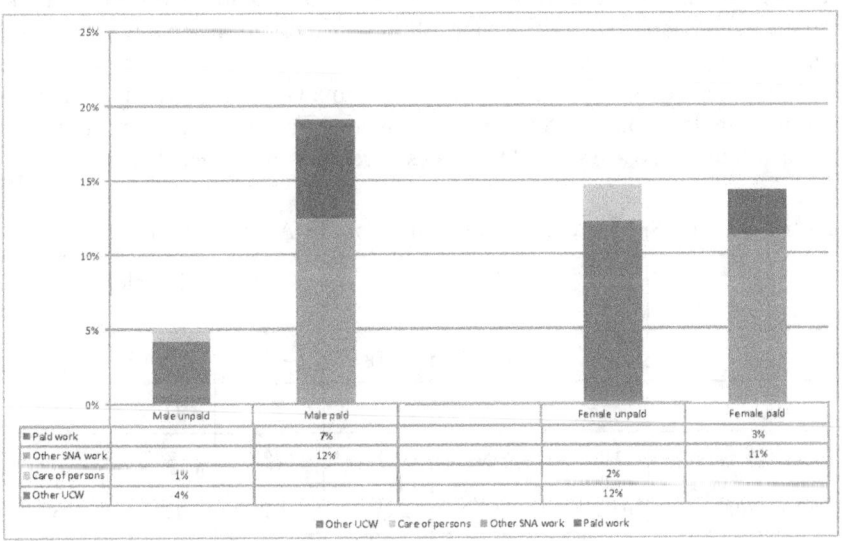

Figure 2.1 Time spent on paid and unpaid work and sex.

females. Care of persons accounts for 1 per cent of the day for the average male, compared to 2 per cent of the day for the average female.

The graph is useful in highlighting once again that care of persons accounts for a small proportion of the unpaid care work done by both females and males, although a larger amount in both proportionate and absolute terms for females than males. Paid work narrowly defined also accounts for a relatively small proportion of the time spent on SNA work, but a larger proportion of SNA time for males and females. Of the time spent on subsistence work, close on 13 per cent is spent on collection of fuel and water. This factor needs to be borne in mind given that colloquially, and even in analysis, most people conceive of these two activities as part of housework. The basic gender differences seen in the preceding tables are expected, and will not be commented on every time in the set of tables that follows.

There are marked differences across age groups in patterns of paid and unpaid work. For both male and female, the 18–49-year-olds tend to spend substantially more of their time on SNA work and the more narrowly defined paid work category than the other groups. Nevertheless, the older men do more SNA work, and also more paid work narrowly defined, than the middle age group of women. Male children spend a tenth of their day on SNA work, while female children spend 8 per cent of the day. Almost all of this is subsistence-type work, including collection of fuel and water. In respect of unpaid work, among females the middle age group again spends more time than others, but this difference does not hold in respect of males. For each age group, males spend noticeably more time on SNA work than on unpaid care work while for women the difference between time spent on unpaid care work and SNA work is small for each of the female age groups. The tables that follow in this section include only those aged 18 years and older.

Table 2.3 shows married men spending somewhat longer than never married (i.e. single) people on SNA and paid work. (The results in respect of widowed and divorced are shaded for males to remind the reader that the samples

Table 2.2 Time Spent on Paid and Unpaid Work by Age Group and Sex

	Male			Female		
	5–17	18–49	50+	5–17	18–49	50+
UCW	5%	5%	5%	9%	19%	14%
Care of persons	1%	1%	1%	1%	3%	2%
SNA work	10%	27%	21%	8%	19%	16%
Paid work	1%	12%	7%	1%	5%	2%

Table 2.3 Time Spent by Adults on Paid and Unpaid Work by Marital Status and Sex

	Male				Female			
	Single	Married	Widowed	Divorced	Single	Married	Widowed	Divorced
UCW	5%	5%	7%	8%	16%	20%	13%	16%
Care of persons	0%	1%	1%	1%	2%	4%	1%	3%
SNA work	24%	26%	16%	25%	18%	18%	16%	20%
Paid work	10%	11%	7%	11%	7%	3%	3%	6%

Table 2.4 Time Spent by Adults on Paid and Unpaid Work by Co-Residence with Young Children and Sex

	Male		Female	
	No children	Children	No children	Children
UCW	5%	5%	15%	20%
Care of persons	0%	1%	1%	4%
SNA work	24%	26%	19%	18%
Paid work	10%	10%	6%	3%

Table 2.5 Time Spent by Adults on Paid and Unpaid Work by Work Status and Sex

	Male			Female		
	Employed	Unemployed	NEA	Employed	Unemployed	NEA
UCW	5%	5%	3%	18%	24%	12%
Care of persons	0%	1%	0%	3%	3%	2%
SNA work	24%	26%	3%	20%	5%	4%
Paid work	10%	10%	0%	5%	1%	1%

are small and the results thus unreliable). For women, the pattern is reversed in respect of paid work while married and single women spend more or less the same amount of time on SNA work. Divorced women tend to spend longer on paid work than married ones. In terms of unpaid work, married women spend longer than all other groups, while there is no noticeable difference between the time spent on unpaid work between married and single men.

The fact that married females tend to spend more time than other groups on unpaid care work might in part reflect the greater likelihood that they will be caring for children. Table 2.4 reveals a five percentage point increase in the amount of unpaid care work done by women, and a three percentage point increase in the proportion of the day spent on care of persons when there is a young child in the household. For men, there is no such effect. Women in households with young children do almost the same amount of SNA work as other women, but less of their work tends to be paid. Among men, those in households with young children tend to do slightly more SNA work than those in other types of households.

Table 2.5 shows that both men and women who are not economically active spend less time, on average, than other men and women on both paid SNA work and unpaid care work. Among both women and men, the unemployed tend to spend more time on unpaid care work than other groups. These findings must be treated with some caution because of the smallish sample sizes but are marked enough to be worth noting. As expected given the definitions, paid work is far more common among employed men and women than among the other groups. The fact that some unemployed people record spending time on paid work could reflect the inclusion, noted previously, of seeking work in the paid work category in terms of the time use classification, under-recording of employment by the standard labour force questions used to classify respondents by work status, and the fact that the week covered by the time use survey was not the same as the reference week for the main ILFS employment questions.

The ILFS questionnaire included, among the relationship codes, one for domestic workers. This information allows us to classify households into two groups—those that have a live-in domestic worker and those that do not. We can then compare the time use patterns of those, other than these domestic workers, who live in each of the two categories of households. Examination of the data shows virtually no difference in time use of men between the two categories of household. For women, those in households without live-in domestic help spend 14 per cent of their day on SNA work, 3 per cent on paid work and 15 per cent on unpaid care work. In contrast, those in households with domestic workers spend 17 per cent of their day on SNA work, 10 per cent on paid work, and 11 per cent on unpaid care work. These patterns suggest that domestic workers help to lighten the unpaid care work load on other females in the household and/or, where women are in paid employment, households are more likely to hire a domestic worker.

Table 2.6 Time Spent by Adults on Paid and Unpaid Work by Educational Achievement Status and Sex

	Male			Female		
	None	Primary	Secondary	None	Primary	Secondary
UCW	5%	5%	5%	16%	19%	16%
Care of persons	1%	1%	1%	3%	3%	2%
SNA work	23%	26%	25%	18%	18%	15%
Paid work	4%	11%	20%	2%	5%	10%

Table 2.7 Time Spent by Adults on Paid and Unpaid Work by Settlement Type and Sex

	Male		Female	
	No children	Children	No children	Children
UCW	5%	5%	18%	19%
Care of persons	1%	1%	3%	3%
SNA work	24%	28%	19%	16%
Paid work	6%	23%	2%	10%

Table 2.8 Time Spent by Adults on Paid and Unpaid Work by Household Income (Tshs 1000) and Sex

	Male				Female			
	<50	59–99	100–199	200+	<50	59–99	100–199	200+
UCW	6%	5%	5%	4%	17%	19%	19%	17%
Care of persons	1%	1%	1%	1%	3%	3%	3%	3%
SNA work	23%	27%	28%	26%	18%	18%	18%	17%
Paid work	6%	14%	17%	16%	3%	5%	7%	8%

Table 2.6 shows a marked increase in the time spent by both men and women on narrowly defined paid work with increasing education. The same pattern is not found in respect of SNA work as a whole. Instead, women with secondary education or more tend to spend less time on SNA work than their less-educated counterparts. In respect of unpaid care work, the patterns are more or less constant for men across all educational groupings. Among adult women, the amount of unpaid care work seems to peak among those with primary education.

Table 2.7 shows urban men spending a higher proportion of their time on SNA and paid work than rural men. The difference is particularly marked in respect of paid work. This reflects the fact that many rural men will be working in subsistence agriculture. Among women, those in rural areas tend to spend longer on SNA work, but less time on paid work. There is little difference between rural and urban areas in the patterns for either women or men in respect of unpaid care work and care of persons.

Table 2.8 shows very little change in time use patterns for either males or females with changes in household income aside from a decrease in the amount of time spent by males on both SNA work and paid work among the poorest households. For SNA work this difference is only evident for the poorest households. For paid work narrowly defined it is evident for both of the two poorest household groupings. This decrease could be part of the reason for the poverty of these households. As with other disaggregations, for each income category, men spend longer on SNA work than on unpaid care work, whereas there is little difference between the time spent by women on the two categories across the income groups. Among men, the time spent on paid work more narrowly defined is greater than time spent on all unpaid care work for all but the poorest group.

Table 2.9 shows that among both women and men, those living in adult-only households tend to spend longer on SNA and paid work than those

Table 2.9 Time Spent on Paid and Unpaid Work by Household Composition and Sex

	Male				Female			
	Ch+Sd	Ch+Ad+Old	Ad	Ch+Old	Ch+Sd	Ch+Ad+Old	Ad	Ch+Old
UCW	5%	5%	6%	5%	20%	16%	16%	16%
Care of persons	1%	1%	1%	1%	4%	3%	0%	1%
SNA work	27%	23%	30%	17%	19%	17%	21%	18%
Paid work	12%	8%	19%	4%	5%	3%	11%	2%

Tanzania 57

in other households, while time spent on this work are among the lowest for households that contain only older people and children. These patterns mainly reflect the fact that older people are less likely than other adults to do SNA and paid work and would thus affect the averages for the non-adult-only households. The patterns are different in respect of unpaid care work. Male engagement changes very little across the different household types. For females, those in households with children and adults tend to spend the longest time on both unpaid care work and care of persons more narrowly defined. The other household types are similar in the amount of unpaid care work, but care of persons accounts for the least time in adult-only households, at less than 1 per cent of the average day.

PREVALENCE OF PERSONAL CARE AND PAID WORK

The set of previous tables yields very small percentages of the day in respect of care of persons, in particular, as well as in respect of paid work for some groupings. One of the main reasons for this is that the percentages are derived from averages across the full grouping. Where only a small proportion of a particular group does a particular type of activity, the average is therefore small for the group as a whole even though particular individuals might be spending fairly substantial amounts of time on these activities.

This section briefly explores the extent to which this fact explains small percentages of time reported before by recording the percentage of males and females that spent any time at all during the seven days covered by the survey on (a) care of persons; (b) the more narrowly defined category of paid work used previously i.e. excluding subsistence-type work and fetching of fuel and water; and (c) both activities. The section also explores the impact on prevalence rates of the fact that the Tanzanian time use survey captured activities over seven days, in that this approach produces higher percentages than surveys that cover fewer days as a person will be recorded as doing an activity even if this was done on only one of the seven days.

Figure 2.2 illustrates the overall male and female patterns for engagement in care of persons, paid work, and both activities in the days covered by the survey. It shows that, overall, 55 per cent of females but only 34 per cent of males spent some time on person care in the previous 24 hours, while 22 per cent of females and 32 per cent of males spent some time on paid work. Only 14 per cent of males and 12 per cent of women did both. If analysis is confined to adults, 65 per cent of females and 38 per cent of males do some care of persons, while 29 per cent and 46 per cent respectively do some paid work. The percentage doing both types of activity is the same for women and men, at 18 per cent.

As noted previously, these percentages are higher than they would be if only one day were covered. To get a sense of how the number of days affects the findings, we calculate the percentage of males and females that did

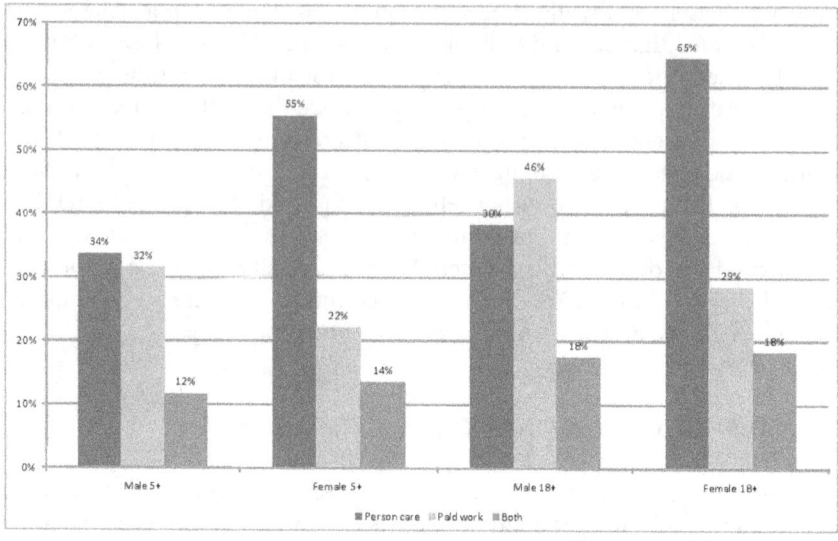

Figure 2.2 Percentage of people doing person care and paid work by sex.

some care of persons every day for which a diary was completed. Participation rates fall to 16 per cent for females and 3 per cent for males, rather than the 55 per cent and 34 per cent previously calculated. If we treat each person-day as a different observation, participations rates are 35 per cent for females and 14 per cent for males. This mimics what might happen in a survey that asked about one random day for each respondent.

EXPLORING CARE OF PERSONS IN MORE DETAIL

This section explores care of persons in more detail. The section uses the full-minute rather than the 24-hour minute and thus captures the full duration of time spent on care work by individuals from different groups. The figures reported in the following paragraphs thus represent minutes rather than the percentage of the day used in an earlier section.

Tanzania elaborated the United Nations' international classification for time use survey by disaggregating the codes relating to care of adults. Separate codes were specified for care of sick, disabled and elderly adults. This was done so that the survey could provide more specific information in relation to the care burden imposed by the HIV and AIDS pandemic, which was one of the motivations for conducting the survey.

Table 2.10 shows the mean time per day recorded for all person care activities, including both activities in category 5 and the three person care activities in category 6. The table includes the full sample, including children. The bold rows indicate codes relating specifically to sick adults. The italic row is for care of adults where it was not clear whether it was for the sick, disabled or elderly. The estimates shown in the table are all—except for physical care of children—very small. This is explained by the relatively low participation rates for most of these activities. The estimates are therefore shown to a decimal place to be able to appreciate smaller differences. Comparison of the bold estimates with those for care of elderly and disabled adults shows that the former are consistently larger than the latter, suggesting that care of the sick is posing more of a burden on Tanzanian society than care of the elderly or care of disabled adults. Nevertheless, codes explicitly naming care of children account for 30.1 minutes for females and 6.9 for males, compared to only 2.6 and 2.3 minutes respectively for codes naming sick adults, 0.1 for both males and females for codes explicitly naming the disabled, and 0.9 minutes for both males and females for codes explicitly naming the elderly.

The analysis that follows distinguishes between a broader measure of "care of persons" and a narrower measure of "active care". The difference between the two is that the latter excludes supervision of those needing care and travel related to care, which are regarded as "passive care". Accompanying children or others is classified as active care as it is relatively difficult to do other activities at the same time.

This analysis confirms the earlier pattern of women in the middle age group bearing the main burden of care of persons, in that women of this age group do 55 minutes of care of persons and 46 minutes of active care compared to 24 and 27 minutes respectively or less for the other age groups. The ratio of active:passive care is also highest for this group, in that 84 per cent of care of persons for women in this age group involves active care, while this is true of 70 per cent of care of persons for women in the other age groups. To simplify the analysis, further discussion of the patterns excludes children.

We again find the highest time for married women. Both married men and married women spend about twice as long on active and passive care as their single counterparts. Divorced women constitute the second most burdened group in terms of both person care in general and active care in particular.

Women co-residing with young children report more than 2 hours on care of persons, and close on 2 hours on active care. Men co-residing with young children spend only 16 minutes per day on average on care of persons, and only ten minutes on active care. There is little difference in the amount of care done by men living in households with young children and women living in households without them.

Those who are not economically active spend less time on care than the employed. One reason for this is that those who have people needing care—whether children, old people or sick people—in the household, are often also forced to earn money to be able to support these dependants.

Table 2.10 Mean Time Spent Per Day on Activities Related to Care of Persons by Sex, 24-hour Minute

Activity	Male	Female
Physical care of children: washing dressing etc	4.4	24.9
Teaching, training and instruction of children	0.2	0.4
Accompanying children to places	0.2	0.2
Waiting to accompany children	0.0	0.0
Physical care of the sick, disabled, elderly	1.1	1.0
Physical care of sick adults	0.8	1.1
Physical care of disabled adults	0.0	0.0
Physical care of elderly adults	0.3	0.4
Accompanying sick adult to receive care	0.1	0.1
Accompanying disabled adult to receive care	0.0	0.0
Accompanying elderly adult to receive care	0.0	0.0
Waiting to accompany adult to receive care	0.0	0.0
Supervising children needing care	1.9	4.3
Supervising sick adult needing care	0.4	0.4
Supervising disabled needing care	0.0	0.1
Supervising elderly needing care	0.2	0.2
Travel related to care of children	0.2	0.3
Travel related to care of sick adult	1.0	1.0
Travel related to care of disabled adult	0.0	0.0
Travel related to care of elderly adult	0.4	0.3
Waiting for travel related to care	0.0	0.0
Other care of children, the sick, elderly & disabled	0.4	0.5
Caring for non-household children	0.0	0.0
Caring for non-household sick adult	0.1	0.0
Caring for non-household elderly adult	0.0	0.0

The pattern holds for both women and men, and for both care of persons in general and active care.

Adults with primary education spend longer on care activities than those with less or more education. The pattern is stronger for women than for men. Less time is spent on care of persons by women in urban than women in rural areas. For men, the amounts of time spent on care are very similar for rural and urban areas.

There is little change in time spent on care with changes in household income except that, as noted previously, women in the wealthiest households tend to spend less time on care than those in poorer households.

Women in child-plus-adult households spend longer on care of persons than those in other types of household. The next highest expenditure of time is found among women living in three-generation households. Among both women and men, time spent on care of persons drops markedly for those living in adult-only households and those in child-plus-older person households.

SUMMARISING THE KEY DETERMINANTS OF TIME SPENT ON CARE

In this section we report the results of Tobit estimations which test the strength of the various relationships shown in the previous tables. For the first estimation we use full minutes (i.e. full duration) of time spent by individuals on care of persons in the household (codes 500–599) as well as care for those in other households (codes 671–674). We regress against being male, being married), being employed, being co-resident with a child under 7 years of age (Childed), living in a rural area, having no schooling, having secondary education or higher (SecondPlus), living in a household containing only child/ren and older people (KidAndOld), living in a household containing only child/ren and middle-aged adult/s (KidAndAdult), being in a 'three-generation' household, being in the poorest groups of households (PoorHH), age and age squared. In terms of household composition, the implicit comparator is an adult-only household. The full sample is included in the estimation so as to capture the full relationship to age.

Table 2.11 confirms that living in a rural area, level of education, most forms of household composition and living in a poorer household are not significant determinants ($P<=0.005$) of time spent on care of persons. Among those that are significant, co-residing with a child has the strongest effect of the dummy variables, closely followed by being male, and then being married and being employed. Being male tends to reduce the time spent on care of persons, while the other factors all increase the time. All the variables combined accounted for 13.9 per cent of the correlation between the fitted values and actual values for time spent on care of persons.

Table 2.11 Estimation Results on Duration of Time Spent on Care of Persons

	Coef.	Std. Err.	t	P>|t|	95% Conf. Interval	
Male	-56.1	2.0	-27.56	0.0000	-60.1	-52.1
Married	32.2	2.7	11.89	0.0000	26.9	37.6
Employed	15.5	2.8	5.53	0.0000	10.0	21.0
Childed	61.1	2.9	21.09	0.0000	55.4	66.8
Rural	1.7	2.4	0.72	0.4720	-2.9	6.3
NoSchooling	2.1	2.4	0.85	0.3930	-2.7	6.9
SecondPlus	-3.6	4.2	-0.86	0.3880	-11.9	4.6
KidAndOld	-2.9	5.8	-0.5	0.6190	-14.2	8.4
KidAndAdult	13.8	4.4	3.16	0.0020	5.2	22.3
ThreeGen	8.4	4.3	1.98	0.0470	0.1	16.8
PoorHH	4.6	2.1	2.21	0.0270	0.5	8.8
Age	1.2	0.3	4.32	0.0000	0.7	1.7
AgeSquared	0.0	0.0	-4.33	0.0000	0.0	0.0
Constant	-92.6	5.5	-16.92	0.0000	-103.3	-81.9

The determinants of care change if we define care broadly to define all types of unpaid care work. Table 2.12 reveals that gender now has the highest coefficient by far among the dummy variables, and the coefficient is much larger than for care more narrowly defined. Being married and being employed are also strong determinants of time spent on unpaid care work. Having no schooling or having secondary schooling and above tends to decrease the amount of unpaid care work done when compared with those with primary schooling. Living in a rural area now has a negative effect on the amount of time spent on unpaid care work, as does living in a household with three generations. Other forms of household composition and living in a poor household do not have a significant effect on the amount of time spent on unpaid care work. All the variables combined accounted for 34.5 per cent of the correlation between the fitted values and actual values for time spent on unpaid care work.

The preceding Tobit estimations confirm that many of the patterns shown in the previous tabulations are statistically significant. The advantage of the Tobit estimations is that they show the relative strength of the different factors, controlling for other factors used in the estimation. Thus, for example, a simple tabulation of time use by sex and marital status can be misleading because some of the pattern of greater time spend on care by

Table 2.12 Estimation Results on Duration of Time Spent on Unpaid Care Work

	Coef.	Std. Err.	t	P>|t|	95% Conf. Interval	
Male	-157.7	2.51	-62.94	0.0000	-162.6	-152.8
Married	36.1	3.48	10.39	0.0000	29.3	43.0
Employed	29.0	3.44	8.43	0.0000	22.3	35.8
Childed	19.6	3.31	5.93	0.0000	13.2	26.1
Rural	-15.2	2.94	-5.19	0.0000	-21.0	-9.5
NoSchooling	-10.7	3.12	-3.43	0.0010	-16.8	-4.6
SecondPlus	-14.6	5.13	-2.84	0.0050	-24.6	-4.5
KidAndOld	0.1	6.53	0.02	0.9820	-12.7	12.9
KidAndAdult	-9.3	4.99	-1.87	0.0620	-19.1	0.5
ThreeGen	-17.9	4.85	-3.69	0.0000	-27.4	-8.4
PoorHH	4.6	2.66	1.72	0.0860	-0.7	9.8
Age	4.1	0.34	12	0.0000	3.4	4.8
AgeSquared	-0.1	0.00	-13.5	0.0000	-0.1	0.0
Constant	140.5	6.48	21.68	0.0000	127.8	153.2

married would be caused by the fact that younger people are less likely to be married, and older people tend to do more care work than younger ones. The estimations, by including both marital status and age, show the effect of each of these separately.

Finally, the Tobit estimations are useful in reminding us that the strength of the influence of different factors on time spent on care depends to some extent on the definition of care used.

EXPLORING BEYOND MEANS

Most of the time estimates presented in this chapter have taken the form of means. Means can be misleading to the extent that they hide the pattern of the distribution of time use. The two figures which follow give some indication of the extent to which the distribution of time spent on unpaid care work and person care is skewed, even among the actors. The figures are based on the full minute, which reflects the full duration of simultaneous activities. The figures reflect the number of minutes spent per day, but these estimates represent an average of the seven day's worth of data collected for each respondent.

64 Debbie Budlender

Figure 2.3 shows that close on 14 per cent of males compared to less than 4 per cent of females spend no time at all on unpaid care work on an average day. The distributions for both male and female are asymmetric, but that for females shows a fairly even distribution across each of the half hours between 30 minutes and 6 hours after which there is a long tail, while for men there is a rapid drop-off. These patterns suggest that males who do UCW do a fairly consistently low amount.

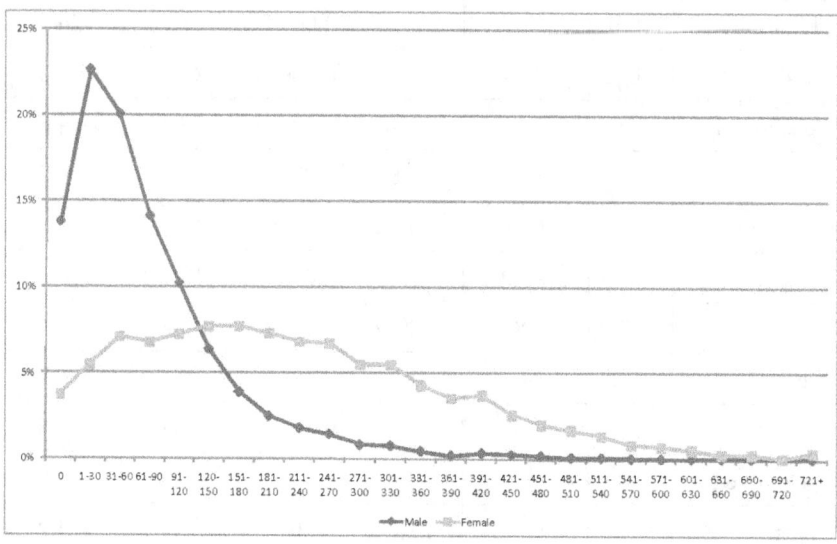

Figure 2.3 Distribution of time spent on unpaid work by sex.

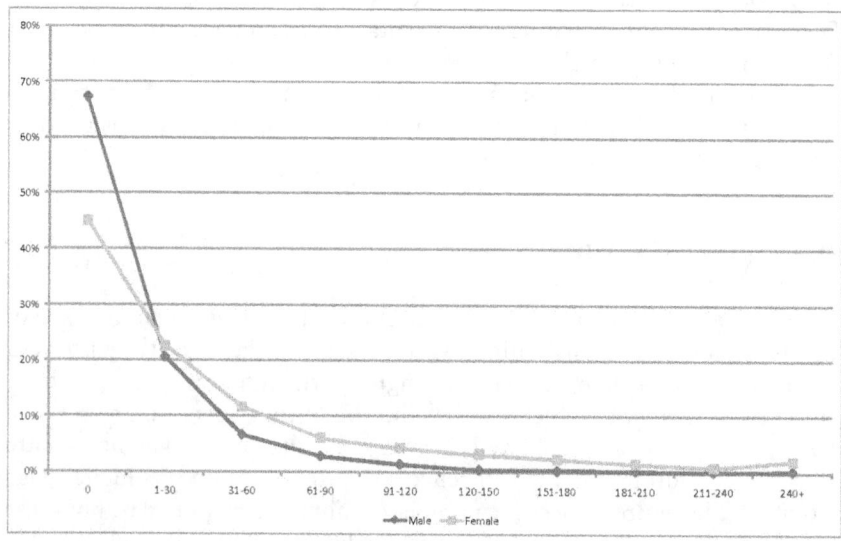

Figure 2.4 Distribution of time spent on person care.

Figure 2.4 shows that 67 per cent of males and 45 per cent of females spend no time on person care on an average day. At the other end of the scale, negligible numbers of males, but 2 per cent of females spend 6 hours or longer on this activity. The figure also shows, as with unpaid care work more generally, a more distinct tail for females than males.

CALCULATING THE VALUE OF UNPAID WORK

In this section we estimate the value, in money terms, of unpaid care work and person. The underlying idea behind the approach is to estimate the number of hours spent on these types of work and multiply this by some measure of hourly earnings.

To get the estimates of earnings, we use data from the ILFS of 2006, the same survey which had time use as a module. A particular challenge in the Tanzanian case is that a large proportion of working people do not report cash earnings. These include the many people whose main work is in subsistence agriculture (64 per cent of employed people are reported to be working on their own farm or *shamba*), and others doing unpaid work in family businesses or agriculture (16 per cent of all employed people) and as domestic workers who might be paid in kind. The proportion of unpaid workers is increased by the fact that the data cover employed children from the age of 5 years. For the valuation, we have used only those who report non-zero earnings. As will be seen, this generates comparative values for unpaid care work and some other macro measures that might seem counter-intuitive. It could be argued that using only non-zero earnings does not provide a true reflection of real "earnings" in the Tanzania labour market. Alternatively, it could be argued that a true valuation, when comparing the value of unpaid care work with that of SNA work, should also impute cash values to the unpaid SNA work.

When using the average wage approach, we include all employed people, whether employees, self-employed or own-account. However, as noted previously, we exclude all those for whom zero earnings or no earnings are recorded. For employees, the ILFS asks about gross cash income, while for non-agricultural self-employment and own account work it asks about net income from the business.

When using the generalist approach, we use weighted (by the number in an occupation) non-zero wages/salaries for a range of different occupations that do work similar to that done in the home. We exclude teachers, despite some care work resembling teaching, because the large number of teachers would skew the weighted average upwards more than the amount of teaching done in most homes would warrant.

A total of 2,704 (unweighted) individuals are recorded across all these categories, of whom 79 per cent are domestic helpers and cleaners. Of concern for our purposes, is that only 444 (16 per cent) of these individuals record non-zero wages.

We calculate the value of both unpaid care work as a whole and of person care. For the first calculation we use categories 4 through 6 of the activity classification, plus collection of fuel and water as these are not currently included in Tanzania's GDP calculations. For person care i.e. category 5 of the activity classification, plus codes 671 through 673 representing care of persons in other households. In estimating the hours, we use the full-minute approach, as this represents the time actually spent on these activities.

In absolute terms the value of unpaid care work is estimated at between Tshs 5,887bn and Tshs 10,521bn, while the value of person care lies somewhere between Tshs 898bn and RTshs 1,601bn. The following sections compare these values with various other measures of the Tanzanian economy of 2006.

For unpaid care work, the percentage which this constitutes of GDP ranges from 35 per cent when using the median generalist wage, to 63 per cent when using median earnings of all earners. For the narrower measure of person care, the value is equivalent to between 5 per cent and 10 per cent of GDP. For both measures, the disaggregated approaches show that the female contribution is far larger than that of males, even though each hour of female work is given a lower value than an equivalent hour of male work. If the overall median was used rather than separate medians for males and females, the median earnings approach would result in unpaid care work being valued at Tshs. 10,904bn, or 66 per cent of GDP.

For the comparison with the value of paid work, we use the same ILFS that we have used for valuation of unpaid care work. This yields annual total employee wages and salaries of Tshs. 2,460,251m, and annual total earnings of all earners of Tshs. 11,999,439m.

The value of unpaid care work is equal to several times more than the value of employee wages and salaries when measured by either of our two approaches, while it accounts for between 49 per cent and 88 per cent of all cash earnings, depending on the approach. The interesting finding in respect of employee wages and salaries is a result of the relatively small proportion of employees among the employed population Tanzania, as well as low or non-existent wages for some. Person care accounts for between 37 per cent and 65 per cent of the value of employee wages and salaries, and between 7 per cent and 13 per cent of the value of all cash earnings.

The first tax comparison is with individual income tax, which was estimated at Tshs. 362.8 bn for 2006–2007.[1] The second comparison is with a composite tax measure that includes individual income tax, income tax on security schemes, corporate tax, payroll tax, tax on property, and value-added tax on domestic goods. The estimated amount for this composite was Tshs. 781.5 bn for 2006/07. The final comparator is domestic revenue, at Tshs. 2,461.0 bn for 2006/07.

The value of unpaid care work using the earnings approach is nearly 30 times that of individual income tax. Person care alone has a value more than four times that of individual income tax using the earnings approach.

Both unpaid care work and person care again have values greater than the composite tax measure whatever approach is used. Using the earning approach, the value of unpaid care work appears to be more than 13 times that of composite tax. Unpaid care work is several times domestic revenue in value whichever valuation approach is used. Person care has a value less than that of domestic revenue, but still amounts to close to two-thirds of domestic revenue using the earnings approach and more than one-third using the generalist approach.

The next comparison is with government expenditure on care-related sectors. For other countries the comparison is made with personnel. For Tanzania the full sector allocation is used. We use the allocations for the education and health sectors for 2006–2007. These stood at Tshs. 891.2 bn and Tshs. 427.4 bn respectively if one includes the allocations to districts.

We find that unpaid care work accounts for close on eight times the value of government health and education expenditure using the earnings approach, and more than four times using the generalist approach. Person care has a value greater than that of government expenditure on these two sectors if we use the earnings approach, and more than two-thirds of the value using the generalist approach.

For the final comparison, we compare the value of unpaid care work with remuneration of paid workers, whether employees or self-employed, in care-related occupations as recorded in the ILFS. The choice of occupations is to some extent subjective as many occupations include both care and non-care work. We therefore make judgements about the weight of the care work. For example, we include primary and pre-primary education teaching professionals but exclude secondary and tertiary teachers on the basis that the latter's work will not involve much care.

The calculations yield total earnings of Tshs. 987,360m per annum. Unpaid care work as valued with the average earnings approach is equivalent to more than ten times the paid care workers' earnings. Using the generalist approach, it is still equal to nearly six times as much as paid workers' earnings. The value of person care is equivalent to between one and one and a half times the value of paid care work in the economy.

CONCLUSION

This chapter has analysed the data from Tanzania's first national time use survey. The analysis has confirmed the basic patterns found in other countries, namely that women tend bear far more of the burden of unpaid care work, as well as of person care, than men do. Unlike some other countries, women's rate of participation SNA work is very similar to that of men, although the time spent on this work tends to be less. The analysis has gone far beyond these broad statements, however, in investigating other personal and household characteristics that influence the amount of time spent by women and men, girls and boys, on person care and unpaid care work. The analysis has also confirmed that broad statements that claim that women and girls do all the unpaid care work in the Tanzanian economy and society are untrue and not helpful for policy-making purposes.

The macro comparisons in the latter part of the paper confirm that the amount of unpaid care work and person care done in the economy is huge. The comparisons are, however, complicated when compared to those done for other countries by the fact that a large amount of the SNA work done in Tanzania is also unpaid. Comparisons of volume of work, using hours, are therefore perhaps more useful in the Tanzanian context than using comparisons based on (imputed) money values.

Whichever numbers we use—whether minutes and hours or shillings—they will not tell us the full story. This chapter therefore needs to be read in conjunction with other analyses which draw on qualitative research and other sources. In addition, the time use data cannot tell us much about activities that are done by a relatively small proportion of the population. The inclusion of separate codes for care of sick adults and care of other adults gives some indications of time use that might be a result of the HIV and AIDS pandemic. The proportion of all Tanzanians who do this work is, however, too small to give clear patterns. The fact that more time seems to be spent on care of sick adults than on care of other adults could well reflect the HIV and AIDS burden.

NOTES

1. Thanks are due to Ruth Carlitz of Haki Elimu for finding the tax-related and sector estimates from 2006–2007 Budget Digest, and 2007–2008 Budget Speech and Budget Estimates.

3 South Africa
When Marriage and the Nuclear Family Are Not the Norm

Debbie Budlender

INTRODUCTION

The 2000 time use survey represented the first time that Statistics South Africa had attempted a time use survey. At the time the survey was conducted, Statistics South Africa estimated the country's population at around 44 million, with just under 36 million people aged 10 years and older, the age group covered by the survey.

The South African time use survey utilised a slightly adapted version of the UN trial classification for time use surveys. This classification has ten one-digit categories, three of which correspond to SNA work, three of which correspond to extended SNA work (or unpaid care work), and four of which correspond to non-work activities. The categories making up unpaid care work are (a) household maintenance, management and shopping for own household; (b) care for children, the sick, elderly and disabled for own household; and (c) community services and help to other households.

DESCRIBING THE SAMPLE POPULATION

In the analysis for this chapter, a standard set of disaggregations was used to explore patterns in time use among different groups, namely population group, age group, marital status, relationship to children, employment status, settlement type, and personal and household income level. All of these were cross-tabulated by sex, given the importance of gender in shaping time use.

Overall, 53 per cent of the weighted sample was female, in line with the overall pattern for this age group in the population. In terms of race, Africans dominate, at over three-quarters of the population and whole-population statistics thus usually mirror the African patterns to a large extent. The Indian group is too small to produce very reliable results.

For age group, three categories are used, representing children (10–17 years), the primary reproductive and productive years (18–49 years) and the ones in which having young children is most likely, and those who are older (50 years and older). For the purposes of this chapter, these groups are referred to as children, younger adults and older adults. The middle group accounts for more than half of the weighted sample.

For marital status, the groupings used are, for the purposes of simplicity, termed "single", "married", "widowed" and "divorced". In reality, the categories are slightly more complex than this in that the married group includes those living together "as husband and wife" even if not formally married, while the divorced categories include those who are separated from partners. The "single" group covers those who have never been married i.e. who are not living together with a partner and have not been separated from, or widowed by, one. A noteworthy feature of the sample population is that over half has never been married. In this respect South Africa differs from many other countries. More restricted tabulations reveal that even if we exclude those under 20 or 30 years, 39 per cent and 20 per cent respectively have never been married.

Status in respect of children is measured in terms of both the age of the children, and whether the children live with the individual. Thus the first category ("7–18 alive") reflects individuals who have at least one biological child aged between 7 and 18 years, but none of these children live with them. The second category ("7–18 with") reflects those who have at least one biological child aged 7–18 years living with them. The third and fourth categories are similar, but defined in relation to children under 7 years old, which corresponds more or less to the pre-school age in South Africa and is also the age when children can be expected to need greater care.

Nearly two-thirds of the respondents claimed to have no biological children, but this could be an undercount in that 12 per cent do not seem to have answered the questions relating to children. This 12 per cent were therefore classified, for lack of data, as not having children. Results for this group must be treated with some caution, but might not skew the data too seriously as two-thirds of these people lived in households which contained no children. The overwhelming majority (86 per cent) of the remainder were never married, which might have been the reason for the fieldworker not asking this question. This would clearly be an error given high rates of childbearing outside marriage in the country.

Lack of children was more common among men than women, reflecting in part the men who might impregnate women but not take further interest in the children produced. The fact that those with children who are living elsewhere account for 8 per cent of the sample population, and 22 per cent of those claiming children reveals the extent to which children and parents are separated in the country. Also noteworthy is that 30 per cent (35 per cent male and 21 per cent female) of those claiming children have never been married.

The distribution in respect of work status can be expected to differ from those found in standard labour force statistics for South Africa because of the inclusion of children from age 10 years. Just over two-fifths of the sample is employed, with half of the males in this situation compared to 37 per cent of females. This gender pattern is balanced by the NEA group, where over half of the females are NEA compared to 43 per cent of the males. The relatively small proportion of the sample that is employed accounts for the fact that the survey shows a relatively low average time spent on SNA work.

Nearly half the sample population lives in urban formal settings, and over a third in deep rural areas, which consist primarily of poverty-stricken apartheid-designated "homelands". The fact that women are somewhat more likely than men to be found in deep rural areas reflects the restrictions placed on the movement of African women during the apartheid years. Also to be borne in mind are the strong racial patterns. In particular, 99 per cent of those in deep rural areas, and 97 per cent in urban informal areas, are African.

The time use questionnaire asks about personal and household income using income categories. Personal income referred to the income accruing directly to a particular person, whatever the source i.e. it was not restricted to earned income. Importantly, it thus included grants such as the old age, child support, disability and foster care grants. Responses of zero income were allowed for this question. Household income referred to all money coming into the household. Responses of zero were not allowed here, on the assumption that all households need to have some amount of money to survive. For the purposes of analysis, these two measures were collapsed in each case into four groups. Unfortunately, the categories precluded the use of equal-sized groups.

About a third of the sample claims to have no personal cash income at all, while another third records an income of less than R500 per month. Only about one-fifth have an income of R1,000 or more. The reported patterns in respect of male and female is as expected given employment patterns and other factors, with substantially more men than women in the highest income group. R1,000 was in 2000 higher than the monthly amount of the old age and disability grants, which are the largest grants, and which from July 2000 stood at R540 per month.

Nearly half of respondents live in households with incomes below R800. This is the level that is meant to be used by many municipalities for distinguishing "indigent" from other households for the purposes of subsidy in respect of water and electricity. The remaining respondents are more or less evenly divided in the two categories R800–R1,799 per month, and R1800 and above. The patterns for male and female are more similar than for personal income, but there is as before a tendency for men to live in better-off households. This reflects, among others, the higher female proportion in the population in the poverty-stricken deep rural areas.

In the analysis, sub-groups which account for 5 per cent or less of the sample population are omitted because of concerns about reliability of findings.

TIME SPENT ON PAID AND UNPAID WORK

The first set of tabulations focuses on the amount of time spent by individuals from different groups on what is often loosely referred to as "paid and unpaid work". To tighten the analysis, and to illustrate the differences resulting from different conceptions, the tables show patterns in respect of two measures of what might loosely be termed "paid work" and two measures of what might loosely be termed "unpaid work".

As previously noted, there are three categories in the activity classification system used in South Africa that together cover SNA work. The following analysis uses all three of these categories as a broad measure of "paid work", and the first and third categories as a narrow measure of "paid work". The measures are not exact because, for example, the first and third categories include unpaid non-agricultural SNA work for establishments or non-establishments respectively. This type of work is, however, less common in South Africa than in many other developing countries. The SNA category also includes time reported as being spent seeking employment. Finally, the inclusion of collection of fuel and water as an SNA activity is theoretically correct, but South Africa does not yet include this activity when estimating gross domestic product.

For the broad measure of unpaid work below all three categories of unpaid care work are used. For the narrow measure, termed "care of persons", only care for children, the sick, elderly and disabled for own household is used. Again, these measures are not exact. For example, the third sub-category of unpaid care work includes care of persons activities that relate to non-household members. Nevertheless, the following analysis should give a good idea of the balance (or lack of it) between paid and unpaid work for different groups.

Table 3.1 shows the division of the average male and female day into the ten main categories of activity. The table shows that just over half of the average day is spent on personal care, which includes sleeping, eating, dressing and similar activities. This helps to explain what may seem relatively low percentages of the day spent on unpaid care work and paid work. In the sample, the inclusion of children from age 10 also helps to explain relatively low amounts of time spent on work when averaged across the sample.

The set of tabulations that follows focuses, as does Table 3.1, on the average time spent by all members of a group on particular categories of activity, with the average calculated over all members, whether or not they engaged in that activity. Later analysis will investigate the extent of involvement of members of particular groups by looking at the number of "actors". The tabulations use the 24-hour minute, i.e. a measure which has the total of activities for any particular person summing exactly to 24 hours. The 24-hour minute undercounts activities which are done simultaneously in that the available time is then divided equally between the simultaneous

Table 3.1 Distribution of Activities Over the Day by Sex

	Male		Female	
Activity category	Minutes	%	Minutes	1%
Establishment work	151	11%	82	6%
Primary productions	26	2%	22	2%
Non-establishment work	13	1%	11	1%
Household maintenance	74	5%	181	13%
Care of persons	4	0%	32	2%
Community services	5	0%	3	0%
Learning	109	8%	96	7%
Social & cultural	218	15%	172	12%
Mass media use	112	8%	105	7%
Personal care	728	51%	732	51%
Total	1439	100%	1437	100%

activities. Later analysis in this report uses a "full-hour" minute which drops the 24-hour limitation and measures full duration. Unpaid care work activities–and personal care in particular–are more likely than SNA work activities to be reported as having been done simultaneously. Thus the ratio of "full minutes" to "24-hour minutes" is between 1.03 and 1.06 for two of the three SNA categories, while it is 1.20 for household care. The analysis which follows will therefore to some extent present different paid:unpaid ratios than what would have been presented if the full minute was used.

Figure 3.1 uses a simple male/female split for the whole population to illustrate how two of the reported categories form subsets of the other two reported categories. Thus the males in the sample spend, on average, 13 per cent of their day on SNA work, which is made up of 11 per cent of the day on "paid work" as defined, and a further 2 per cent on subsistence-type work. In contrast, women spend 9 per cent of their day on SNA work, which is made up of 7 per cent on "paid work" and 2 per cent on subsistence-type work. In respect of unpaid work, males spent a total of 6 per cent (the graph does not sum to 6 per cent because of rounding) on unpaid care work, compared to 15 per cent for females. Care of persons accounts

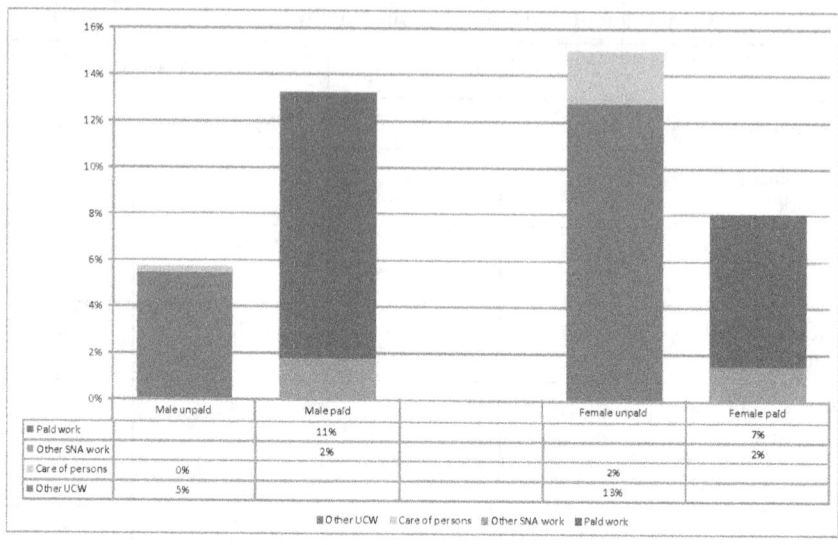

Figure 3.1 Time spent on paid and unpaid work by sex.

for less than half of one per cent of the day for the average male, compared to 2 per cent of the day for the average female.

The graph is useful in highlighting, at the outset, that care of persons accounts for a small proportion of the unpaid care work done by both women and men, although a larger amount in both proportionate and absolute terms for women than men. "Paid work", in contrast, accounts for the majority of time spent on SNA work in South Africa for both women and men, but a larger proportion of SNA time of women than men is spent on subsistence type work. In particular, the time use survey finds 13 per cent of all females compared to 7 per cent of all males reporting collection of water in the last 24 hours, and 5 per cent of all females compared to 2 per cent of all males reporting collection of fuel. The time spent by those who did the activity also tended to be longer for females than males, accounting for 175 and 155 minutes on average respectively for the two activities combined. This factor needs to be borne in mind given that colloquially, and even in analysis, most people conceive of these two activities as part of housework. The basic gender differences seen in the preceding tables are expected, and will not be commented on each time in the set of tables that follows.

Table 3.2 shows white males and females spending a greater proportion of their day on both SNA and paid work than the other groups. (The "of which" in the care of persons and paid work rows reminds the reader that these numbers and percentages are sub-components of unpaid care work and SNA work respectively. "Of which" is omitted in later tables for the sake of simplicity.) The patterns largely reflect the higher employment rates and lower unemployment rates among white people. For each population group, men—as expected—tend to spend more of their day than women on both paid and SNA work. African women and men have the largest proportionate "gap" between SNA work and paid work, reflecting the fact that it is individuals from this group that are more likely to do subsistence work and collection of fuel and water. (The table suggests that this gap is bigger than it is in reality for white men as a result of rounding. Thus, if a decimal place is added, SNA accounts for 18.8 per cent of this sub-group's time compared to the 18.4 per cent of time spent on paid work.)

Among men, there is very little difference across the groups in terms of unpaid work. In contrast, among women, Africans tend to spend a greater proportion of their time on unpaid care work. But the proportion spent on care of persons is more or less constant across the population groups.

Table 3.3 shows, as expected, marked differences across age groups. Among both women and men, the 18–49 year olds tend to spend substantially more of their time on SNA work and the sub-category of SNA work than the other groups. The children—fortunately—are found to spend a very small proportion of time on SNA work, and the fact that most of this

Table 3.2 Time Spent on Paid and Unpaid Work by Population Group and Sex

	Male			Female		
	African	Coloured	Whites	African	Coloured	White
UCW	6%	5%	6%	16%	13%	14%
Care of persons	0%	0%	1%	2%	2%	2%
SNA work	12%	14%	19%	7%	9%	12%
Paid work	10%	14%	18%	5%	9%	12%

Table 3.3 Time Spent on Paid and Unpaid Work by Age Group and Sex

	Male			Female		
	10–17	18–49	50+	10–17	18–49	50+
UCW	4%	6%	7%	8%	18%	15%
Care of persons	0%	0%	0%	1%	3%	1%
SNA work	3%	19%	13%	2%	11%	8%
Paid work	1%	17%	11%	0%	9%	6%

is not paid work suggests that much of it involves collection of fuel and water. The difference between the age groups is less marked for females than for males. In respect of unpaid work, among women the middle age group again spends more time than others, but this difference does not hold in respect of males.

Table 3.4 shows married women and men spending longer than those who are never married on paid work. The same pattern holds for women in respect of unpaid work, but holds very weakly, if at all, for men. The patterns in respect of paid work are influenced by the fact that most of the children are in the "single" category. If children are excluded, SNA work increases to 13 per cent of the day for men and 9 per cent for women, while the narrower category of paid work increases to 12 per cent and 7 per cent respectively. The inclusion of children does not explain, though, why single and married males have very similar patterns in respect of unpaid care work, while married females tend to do significantly more of this work than single ones.

The fact that married females tend to spend more time than other groups on unpaid care work might in part reflect the greater likelihood that they will be caring for children. Table 3.5 zeroes in on this element by comparing the patterns for those with no reported children and those with children between the ages of 7 and 18 years, and those with children under 7 years of age living with them. The table records women with children under 7 years co-resident spending an average of 7 per cent of their day on care of persons, and nearly one quarter of their day on unpaid care work. Interestingly, these women nevertheless tend to spend more of their time on SNA work than those with no reported children. Women with children under 18 years living with them spend noticeably less time on care of persons than those with younger children, and also less time on unpaid care work. They nevertheless spend noticeably more time on unpaid care work than those without children, and more time on paid work than either of the other two groups. The difference in time spent on unpaid care work between women with older and younger children is the same as the difference in time spent on the care of persons between these two groups. This suggests that younger

Table 3.4 Time Spent on Paid and Unpaid Work by Marital Status

	Male		Female	
	Single	Married	Single	Married
UCW	5%	6%	13%	20%
Care of persons	0%	0%	2%	3%
SNA work	8%	22%	6%	11%
Paid work	6%	20%	4%	10%

children do not create a greater need for household chores than older children. Nevertheless, comparison of the total amount of unpaid care work done by women with and without children suggests that children in general do increase the need for housework. Among men, there is very little change in the pattern of unpaid care work with differences in childed status, but men with children living with them tend to spend much more time doing SNA work than those without children.

The patterns for both male and female in respect of those without children are to some extent biased by the fact that children themselves will fall in this category. If children are excluded, there is little difference in unpaid care work for males, but SNA work and paid work increase to 13 per cent and 11 per cent respectively. For females, excluding children results in unpaid care work as a whole increasing from 11 per cent to 14 per cent, while SNA work increases to 9 per cent and paid work to 7 per cent. Excluding children thus results in the same overall pattern of those without children doing noticeably less care work than those who have children living with them. Among men, this group also does noticeably less paid work, but this pattern is less evident for women.

Table 3.5 Time Spent on Paid and Unpaid Work by Child Status and Sex

	Male			Female		
	No children	7-18 with	<7 with	No children	7-18 with	<7 with
UCW	6%	7%	6%	11%	18%	23%
Care of persons	0%	1%	1%	1%	2%	7%
SNA work	8%	21%	26%	6%	13%	10%
Paid work	6%	19%	24%	4%	11%	8%

Table 3.6 Time Spent on Paid and Unpaid Work by Work Status and Sex

	Male			Female		
	Employed	Unemployed	NEA	Employed	Unemployed	NEA
UCW	6%	5%	6%	16%	13%	14%
Care of persons	0%	0%	1%	2%	2%	2%
SNA work	12%	14%	19%	7%	9%	12%
Paid work	10%	14%	18%	5%	9%	12%

Table 3.6 shows both men and women who are not economically active (NEA) spending less time, on average, than other men and women on both paid SNA work and unpaid care work. The difference in respect of unpaid care work for NEA and employed women is, however, relatively small. Nevertheless, among both women and men, the unemployed tend to spend more time on unpaid care work than other groups. The same holds strongly in respect of care of persons for women, but not for men. As expected given the definitions, paid work is far more common among employed men and women than among the other groups. The fact that unemployed men record spending an average of 7 per cent of the previous day on paid work could reflect both the inclusion, noted previously, of seeking work in the paid work category in terms of the time use classification, and under-recording of employment by the standard labour force questions used to classify respondents by work status.

The much longer time spent by unemployed women, compared to women who are employed, on unpaid work cannot be explained by a greater tendency to have domestic workers employed in households of employed women in that there is only a small difference in this respect. Thus 6 per cent of unemployed women, compared to 8 per cent of employed women, are living in households where someone who is not a household member (usually a domestic worker) is responsible for most of the housework. This pattern is, in fact, more marked for men, where 3 per cent of unemployed men but 7 per cent of employed men are likely to have a domestic worker working in their home.

Table 3.7 shows noticeably lower proportions of time spent on SNA and paid work by men in deep rural areas when compared to men elsewhere. The same pattern is not found in respect of SNA work for women but is found for paid work. The difference in the pattern for SNA and paid work for women would presumably be accounted for by both engagement in subsistence agriculture and fetching of fuel and water. Another difference between women and men is that the average amount of time spent on SNA and paid work does not differ for men between urban formal and informal areas, while for women it is lower among those living in urban informal

Table 3.7 Time Spent on Paid and Unpaid Work by Settlement Type and Sex

	Male			Female		
	Urban-formal	Urban-informal	Deep-rural	Urban-formal	Urban-informal	Deep-rural
UCW	5%	7%	6%	14%	17%	16%
Care of persons	0%	0%	0%	2%	3%	2%
SNA work	14%	5%	9%	9%	7%	7%
Paid work	4%	14%	5%	9%	7%	3%

areas. For both women and men, there is very little difference in patterns across settlement types in terms of unpaid care work and care of persons.

Table 3.8 shows, as seems logical, that those with higher personal incomes tend to spend a greater proportion of their day on SNA and paid work. What is interesting is that women spend a lower proportion of their day on these types of work than men with the same level of personal income. The proportion of time spent by women and men on unpaid care work and care of persons seems to change very little with personal income, although women in the highest bracket spend less time than others. If we confine the analysis to those with personal incomes of R5,000 or more, women spend an average of 23 per cent of their time on paid SNA work, while unpaid care work drops a further percentage point to 12 per cent. These trends could reflect the ability of these women to pay others to do this work. Among men, in contrast, unpaid care work and person care each increase by one percentage point while the pattern in respect of SNA and paid work remains the same.

Table 3.9 shows a clearer pattern of unpaid care work by women decreasing with increasing household income. The likelihood of this reflecting employment of a domestic worker is borne out by the fact that 17 per cent of households participating in the survey which had incomes of R1,800 or more reported that a person who was not a member of the household bore the main responsibility for housework. Among all other income groups, the percentage was 3 per cent or less. (There are further race patterns, in that only 4 per cent of African and coloured* respondents from households in the highest income bracket appeared to have a domestic worker, compared to 50 per cent of white respondents.) In contrast to the situation for unpaid work, the average time spent by women on SNA and paid work increases

Table 3.8 Time Spent on Paid and Unpaid Work by Personal Income and Sex

	Male				Female			
	No cash	1–500	501–1000	1000+	No cash	1–500	501–1000	1000+
UCW	5%	6%	6%	5%	15%	18%	16%	13%
Care of persons	0%	0%	0%	0%	2%	3%	7%	2%
SNA work	4%	10%	18%	26%	3%	7%	10%	20%
Paid work	2%	8%	16%	26%	1%	6%	8%	20%

*During the apartheid years, every individual was designated as belonging to one of four groups, namely African, coloured, Indian/Asian and white. These categories continue to be used in analysis as a way of assessing the extent to which the legacy of apartheid persists in socio-economic and other terms.

Table 3.9 Time Spent on Paid and Unpaid Work by Household Income and Sex

	Male				Female			
	0–399	400–799	800–1799	1800+	0–399	400–799	800–1799	1800+
UCW	6%	6%	6%	6%	17%	16%	15%	13%
Care of persons	0%	0%	0%	0%	3%	2%	2%	2%
SNA work	11%	9%	15%	16%	7%	6%	7%	12%
Paid work	8%	7%	13%	16%	5%	3%	6%	11%

with increasing income. This is particularly marked for those living in households with incomes of R1,800 or more per month. Among men, the marked increase in time spent on SNA and paid work happens at the lower level, of R800 per month. Men's engagement in unpaid care work does not seem to be affected by household income.

PREVALENCE OF PERSON CARE AND PAID WORK

The set of previous tables yields very small percentages of the day in respect of care of persons, in particular, as well as in respect of paid work for some groupings. One of the main reasons for this is that the percentages are derived from averages across the full grouping. Where only a small proportion of a particular group does a particular type of activity, the average is therefore small for the group as a whole even though particular individuals might be spending fairly substantial amounts of time on these activities.

The difference in the means for the full population and for "actors", i.e. those individuals who did a specified activity in the last 24 hours, can be substantial. For example, if we examine care of persons, including the three activities in respect of persons from other households, mean minutes for males increases from 4 to 72 when changing from the full population to only those who did this activity. Mean minutes for females increases from 40 to 133. The much larger relative increase for males is explained by the relatively low participation rate. Nevertheless, females still work substantially more hours than males on either measure.

Figure 3.2 illustrates the overall male and female patterns for engagement in care of persons, paid work, and both activities in the previous 24 hours. It shows that, overall, 30 per cent of females but only 6 per cent of males spent some time on person care in the previous 24 hours, while 23 per cent of females and 34 per cent of males spent some time on paid work. Only 3 per cent of males and 7 per cent of women did both. In Figure 3.1, the mean time, averaged across the population, of males on person care

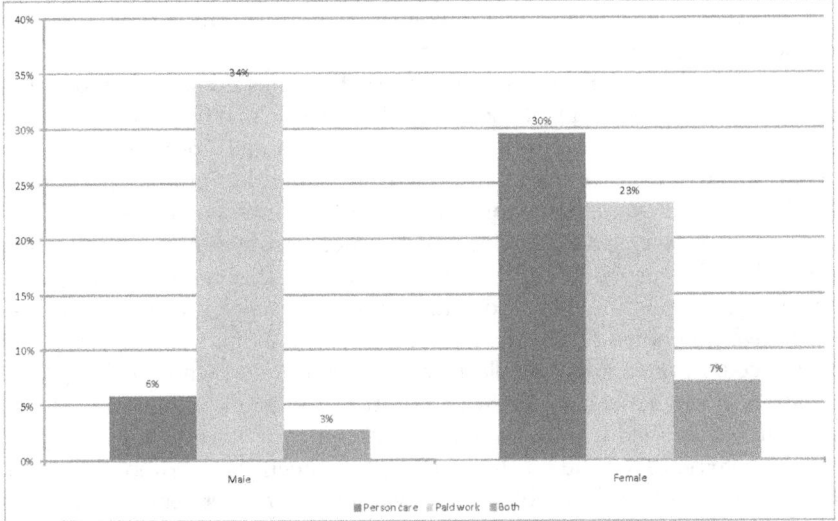

Figure 3.2 Percentage of people doing person care and paid work by sex.

was 0 minutes while that on paid work was 11 minutes. For females the comparable estimates were 2 minutes and 7 minutes.

Across all population groups, females were more likely than males to do some person care and less likely to do paid work. The differences between male and female in respect of person care were more marked for Africans and coloureds than for whites. White men were noticeably more likely than others to do this work, while coloured females were more likely than other females to do so. In respect of paid work, the engagement rates were much higher for whites than for the other population groups, while Africans were lowest. These patterns match the respective employment and unemployment rates. Combining person care and paid work in the same day was most common for white women, and more common for white men than African women. African women were nevertheless six times more likely than African men to combine these two types of work as only 1 per cent of African men recorded doing both types of work in the previous day.

In terms of age group, 41 per cent of females in the prime age group, but only 7 per cent of males, did some person care on the previous day. Among older people, the percentages are 21 per cent and 5 per cent. The percentage of children doing person care is lower than for other groups, but girls were more than three times as likely to do this work as boys. For paid work, about half of males and a third of females in the prime group were active in the past 24 hours, with lower but still substantial rates among the older people. Unlike for the older age groups, there is no gender difference in respect of engagement in paid work among children. Virtually no children did both types of work. Combining the two types of work was most common for women aged 18–49 years. These women were nearly three times as likely as their male counterparts to combine the two types of work.

Over four in ten (43 per cent) of married females do some person care, compared to 23 per cent of those who have never married. For males the prevalence of person care is, as usual, much lower at 10 per cent and 3 per cent respectively. More than half of married males, but only 21 per cent of single males did some paid work in the last 24 hours. For females the percentages are lower, and the relative difference between married and single is smaller. This probably reflects, in part, the fact that many single women are bringing up children without the father's presence (or assistance) and thus have no choice but to do some paid work. Woman also account for 88 per cent of the adults (people aged 18 years or over) who are living with children in the household but with no other adults. Over one in eight (13 per cent) of married women combined both types of work, while only 6 per cent of married men did so. Among single women the likelihood of combining paid work and care of persons was lower, at 4 per cent, but this was about four times the prevalence for single men.

As expected, the likelihood of doing person care increases noticeably with the presence of children. For women, this phenomenon is particularly strong when there are children under 7 years of age. Thus nearly three-quarters of women with young children living with them recorded some care of persons for the previous day. Among men, the likelihood of doing paid work increases when the man has a child living with him, and even further when the child is young. For women, the likelihood increases when the woman has children, but is lower for women with younger children than for those with older children. Finally, 9–10 per cent of men with children living with them did both paid work and care of persons in the previous 24 hours, while this was the case for 19 per cent of women with young children, and 11 per cent of women with older children.

Again as expected, a markedly greater proportion of employed than unemployed or not economically active persons did some paid work in the previous 24 hours. The fact that some unemployed and NEA persons are recorded as doing paid work would reflect both work-seeking (because this is included in the category of SNA work in the activity classification system) and under-recording of employment—especially marginal employment—when using the standard labour force questions. Among men, unemployment and NEA are less likely than employed people to do person care. The same pattern holds for NEA women, but definitely not for unemployed. Only 5 per cent of employed men, and even fewer in other work status groups, did both types of work on the previous day, while this was the case for 16 per cent of employed women.

The survey suggests similar levels of engagement in paid work by men in formal and informal urban areas, but much lower in deep rural areas. Among women, the level is also lowest in deep rural areas, where paid employment opportunities are scarce. But women in informal urban areas are also somewhat less likely than those in formal urban areas to have paid work. For care of persons, there are only small differences for women across the different settlement types, while for men, levels of this type of work are noticeably lower in deep rural areas than elsewhere. The group that is most likely to combine paid work and care of persons is women in formal urban areas.

There is, as might be expected, a clear increase in the prevalence of paid work among both women and men as personal income increases. Among men, the same pattern holds, although more muted, in respect of care of persons, but among women there is no clear pattern. Females with personal income of R1,000 or more per month are, by a large margin, the group with the highest tendency to combine care of persons and paid work. One-fifth (20 per cent) of individuals in this group combine the two types of work, compared to 7 per cent or less in all other groups.

There is also an increasing tendency for women and men to do paid work with increases in household income. For both, however, a higher proportion of those in the lowest income group do paid work than in the next highest income group. This could reflect the fact that the second income group would capture households that are reliant only on a state old age pension. Among men, those in the highest income bracket are markedly more likely than others to do some care of persons. Among women, the pattern fluctuates, but it is those in the poorest group who are most likely to report care of persons.

EXPLORING CARE OF PERSONS IN MORE DETAIL

This section explores care of persons in more detail. It goes beyond participation rates to examine the time spent on this form of care. It uses the "full-minute" rather than the 24-hour minute and thus captures the full duration of time spent on care work by individuals from different groups. In this section the category of person care is refined by adding the three codes relating to care of persons from other households, and the averages are calculated across all individuals in a particular group rather than only for "actors".

The difference between care of persons and active care is that the latter excludes supervision of those needing care. Accompanying children or others is classified as active care as it is relatively difficult to do other activities at the same time. Travel that is not reported as accompaniment is classified as passive care.

We find coloured women (at 43 minutes) spending more time than African (40) and white (37) women, while African men (3 minutes) spend less than other men (8–9 minutes). The difference between the patterns for care of person and active care suggest that white women were somewhat more likely than others to report more passive forms of care such as supervision. Women do significantly more than men of both types of care.

In terms of age, the analysis confirms the earlier pattern of women in the middle age group bearing the main burden of care of persons. These women spend an average of 58 minutes per day on care of persons, as compared to only 24 minutes for the older group and only 10 minutes for the children. Half of the already limited time reported by men in this age group consists of passive care.

For both care of persons as a whole and active care married women tend to spend almost twice as long as single women. In gender terms, the difference in time spent is particularly marked for single women and men.

Women with children under 7 years old reporting nearly 2 hours on care of persons, and more than an hour and a half on active care. Women with older children living with them record just over a half-hour on care of persons, and 24 minutes on active care. Men with young children spend only ten minutes on average on care of persons, and an even lower seven minutes on active care.

Among both women and men, the unemployed record longer time spent on care of persons and active care. But for men this amounts to only eight minutes on care of persons on average. Among women, those in the other work status groups all record over half an hours on average on care of persons, and about half an hour on active care.

Less time is spent on care of persons by women in formal urban settings, with little difference between the other two settlement types. The pattern is different for men, but the average number of minutes is very small for all male groups.

There is no clear pattern in respect of personal income for women. For men, more time is recorded for the highest-earning group in respect of both care of persons and active care. When we turn to household income, we find that women in the poorest households spend longer on care of persons than those in better-off households. There is, however, little difference between the three other income groups. Among men, if anything time spent on care of persons again increases with household income.

SUMMARISING THE KEY DETERMINANTS OF TIME SPENT ON CARE

Finally, we run a Tobit estimation to test the strength of the various relationships shown previously through tables. For this estimation we use "full" minutes (i.e. full duration) of time spent by individuals on care of persons in the household (codes 500–599) as well as care for those in other households (codes 671–673). We regress against being male, being married, being employed, having a child under 7 years living in the household (Childed), being white, falling in the highest household income bracket (HiIncome), years of schooling (HighestEd), age and age squared.

Table 3.10 confirms that all of these factors except race, household income and marital status are significant ($P \leq 0.005$) determinants of time spent on care of persons. Among the dummy factors, having one's young child co-residing has the strongest effect, followed by gender. Being employed also has a marked effect. Being male and being employed tends to reduce the time spent on care of persons, while the other factors all increase the time spent. The aforementioned variables combined account for 18.7 per cent

Table 3.10 Regression Results on Duration of Time Spent on Care

	Coef.	Std. Err.	t	P>t	95% Conf. Interval	
Male	-195.4	6.6	-28.71	0.0000	-208.3	-182.5
Married	15.5	6.2	2.01	0.0450	0.3	24.7
Employed	-43.7	5.8	-7.51	0.0000	-55.1	-32.3
Childed	255.2	6.5	39.16	0.0000	242.4	268.0
White	-0.6	9.8	-0.06	0.9550	-19.8	18.7
High Income	11.4	7.1	1.62	0.1050	-2.4	25.3
HighestEd	2.4	0.8	3.05	0.0020	0.8	3.9
Age	4.1	0.8	4.99	0.0000	2.5	5.7
Age Squared	0.0	0.0	-4.73	0.0000	0.1	0.0
Constant	-264.6	14.7	-18.01	0.0000	-293.4	-235.9

Table 3.11 Regression Results on Duration of Time Spent on Unpaid Care Work

	Coef.	Std. Err.	t	P>t	95% Conf. Interval	
Male	-172.1	3.2	-53.6	0.0000	-178.4	-165.8
Married	5.8	3.9	1.48	0.1380	-1.9	13.4
Employed	-72.4	3.6	-20.19	0.0000	-79.4	-65.4
Childed	91.5	4.3	21.43	0.0000	83.1	99.9
White	-21.2	9.0	-3.52	0.0000	-33.0	-9.4
High Income	-35.9	4.3	-8.31	0.0000	-44.4	-27.4
HighestEd	4.0	0.5	8.57	0.0000	3.1	4.9
Age	10.9	0.5	23.6	0.0000	10.0	11.8
Age Squared	-0.1	0.0	-21.11	0.0000	-0.1	-0.1
Constant	36.8	7.7	4.79	0.0000	-21.8	51.9

86 *Debbie Budlender*

of the variation in the amount of time spent by a particular individual on person care.

The determinants of care change if we define care broadly to define all types of unpaid care work. Table 3.11 reveals that gender now has the highest coefficient among the dummy variables. The effect of the presence of the person's child in the household is at second place, but with a lower coefficient than before. Race and household income become significant determinants, with whites and those in the wealthiest households less likely than others to do this work. The coefficient for age is positive, while that for age squared is negative. This reflects the fact that the likelihood of doing unpaid care work tends to increase with age, but tails off at older ages. Marriage is now the only factor which is not significant. All the other factors together account for about 28.9 per cent of the variation in time spent doing unpaid care work by particular individuals.

EXPLORING BEYOND THE MEANS

Most of the time estimates presented in this chapter take the form of means. Means can be misleading to the extent that they hide the pattern of the distribution of time use. The two figures which follow give some indication of the extent to which the distribution of time spent on unpaid care work and person care is skewed, even among the actors. The figures are based on the full minute, which reflects the full duration of simultaneous activities.

Figure 3.3 shows that close to 30 per cent of males compared to less than 10 per cent of females spent no time at all on unpaid care work on the

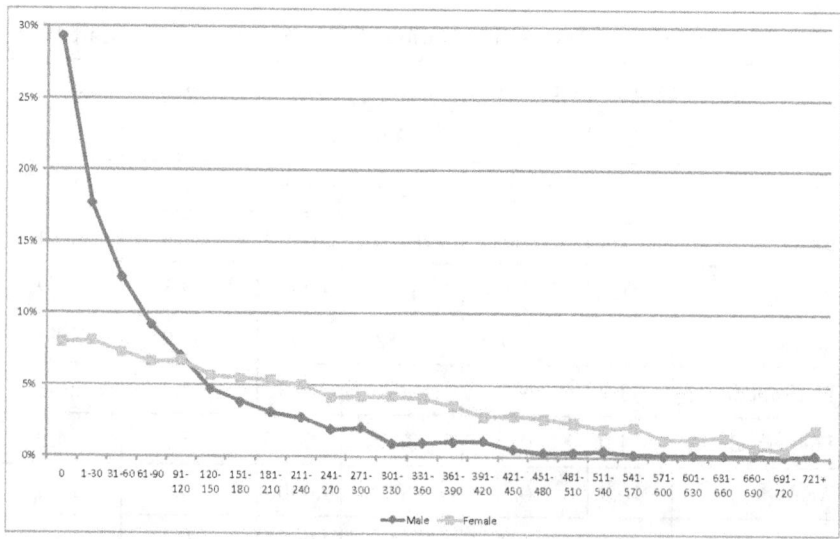

Figure 3.3 Distribution of time spent on unpaid care work by sex.

previous day. At the other end of the scale, a negligible number of males, but 2 per cent of women, spent longer than 12 hours on unpaid care work.

The distributions for both male and female are asymmetric and clearly not normal distributions, but the distribution for women has an extremely long tail, while the distribution for men has a short tail. The short tail for males suggests a low variability i.e. that males do a fairly consistently low amount of UCW. The long tail for women suggests the opposite— high variability and, as a consequence, a notable level of inequality. The high variability confirms that a point estimate, such as the overall mean or median, can mislead, particularly in respect of females, as there is substantial in-group inequality.

Figure 3.4 shows that 94 per cent of males and 70 per cent of females spent no time on person care in the previous day. At the other end of the scale, negligible numbers of males, but 4 per cent of females spent six hours or longer on this activity. The main message from this figure is that most people do not do direct care. The figure also shows, as with unpaid care work more generally, a more distinct tail for females than males.

MACRO MEASURES

In this section we calculate five different macro measures which are intended to give an idea of the size of the care economy relative to other parts of the economy. To make this comparison possible, we first have to assign a monetary value to unpaid care work. We do this by estimating the number of hours worked and multiplying this by some measure of hourly earnings.

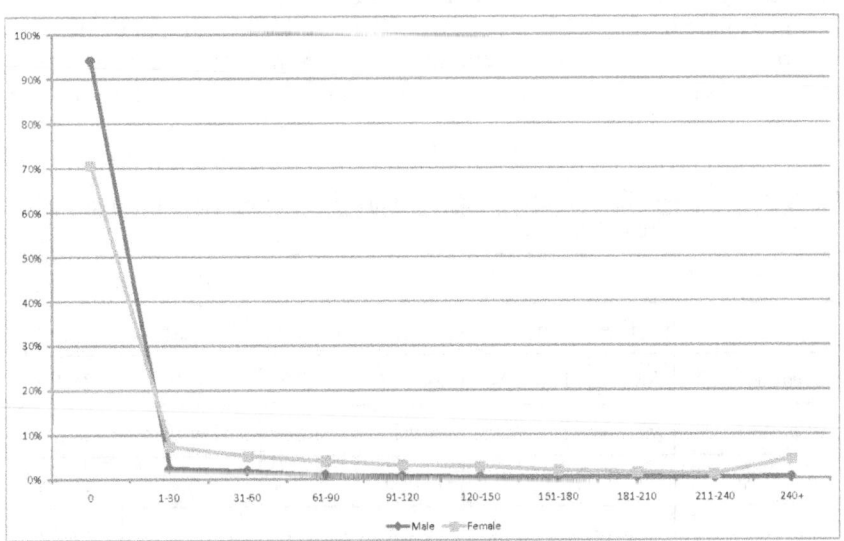

Figure 3.4 Distribution of time spent on person care.

For the purposes of this chapter we use two approaches—the average earnings approach and the generalist approach. Both of these tend to result in lower value estimates than the opportunity cost and specialist approaches. A further choice which results in lower estimates is that we have chosen to use median earnings rather than mean earnings for the averages. In addition, we acknowledge that the estimates of earnings, derived from the labour force survey (LFS) of September 2000 will, as in other countries reflect reported earnings that—as in other countries (Deaton 2003: 8) are often substantially lower than actual earnings. Adjustments for this are not effected in this chapter because of the difficulty of knowing the correct adjustment.

When using the average wage approach, we include all employed people, whether employees, self-employed or own-account. We exclude only those for whom zero earnings or no earnings are recorded. When using the generalist approach, we include two options. For the first option, we use weighted (by the number in an occupation) wages/salaries for a range of different occupations that do work similar to that done in the home. For the second option, we use wages/salaries recorded for all domestic workers (occupational code 9131).

We estimate value for both unpaid care work as a whole and for person care. The latter is defined as category 5 of the activity classification, plus codes 671 through 673 representing care of persons in other households. In estimating the hours, we use the full-minute approach, as this represents the time actually spent on these activities. Our calculations produce an estimate of 586 hours per year spent on unpaid care work by the average male as opposed to 1,569 hours by the average female. For person care the comparable estimates are 27 hours and 242 hours.

In absolute terms, Table 3.12 reveals that the value of unpaid care work is estimated at between R96.72bn and R269.75bn, while the value of person care lies somewhere between R12.32bn and R33.15bn. These estimates

Table 3.12 Total Value of Unpaid Care Work and Person Care Per Year (Rbn): Different Approaches

	UCW			Person		
	Male	Female	Total	Male	Female	Total
All earners	78.54	170.60	249.14	3.59	26.30	29.89
All employees	77.83	191.92	269.75	3.56	29.58	33.15
Generalist			130.20			16.58
Domestic worker			96.72			12.32

can then be compared with various other measures of the South African economy of 2000.

Calculated as a percentage of total GDP, for unpaid care work, the percentage ranges from 30.4 per cent when using the median wage for all employees, to 10.9 per cent when using the median wage of domestic workers. This large difference reflects the very low wages paid to domestic workers in South Africa, exacerbated by the fact that there was no minimum wage for domestic workers in 2000. For the narrower measure of person care, the value is equivalent to between 1.4 per cent and 3.7 per cent of GDP. For both measures, the disaggregated approaches show that the female contribution is far larger than that of males, even though each hour of female work is given a lower value than an equivalent hour of male work.

For the comparison with the value of paid work, we use the same LFS that we have used for valuation of unpaid care work. Unpaid care work is found to be equivalent to somewhere between 19 per cent and 53 per cent of the value of paid work, depending on the approach used for valuation. For person care, the respective minimum and maximum percentages are 2 per cent and 7 per cent. For men, unpaid care work is equivalent to less than a quarter of the value of paid work, while for women the value of unpaid care work is much the same as that of paid work despite the lower earnings used in the valuation.

For the tax comparison we use two different measures for the 2000/01 financial year. The first measure is that for personal and individual tax, in the amount of R86,478.0m. The second is total gross tax, in the amount of R220,334.2m (National Treasury 2003a: 198). Of this amount, R86,478 was sourced from personal direct income tax.

The value of unpaid care work thus clearly exceeds that of personal tax, whatever approach to valuation is adopted. For two approaches, the value of unpaid care work even exceeds total tax. Person care alone accounts for more than a third of the value of personal tax using two measures.

In South Africa, social services such as education, health and social welfare are primarily delivered by the provincial sphere of government. For the comparison with government social services we therefore aggregate the personnel expenditure of the national and provincial departments of education (R39,308m), health (R16,408m) and social development (R921m) (National Treasury 2003b: 57; 78; 97) to arrive at a total estimate of social services personnel expenditure of R56,637m for the 2000/01 financial year. (Social development is similar to the sector described as (social) welfare in many other countries.) This value is an over-estimate to the extent that it includes administrative and managerial staff. It is an under-estimate to the extent that it excludes the salaries of services that are contracted out or subsidised, including grant delivery and a range of social welfare services performed by non-governmental organisations.

Our calculations suggest that the value of unpaid care work could be more than four times that of government's social services. Even on the modest measure based on domestic worker wages, the value is nearly double that of the social services spending on personnel. Person care accounts for more than half of the value of government social services using two valuation approaches, and close to a quarter of the value using the most modest measure.

For the final comparison, we compare the value of unpaid care work with remuneration of paid workers in care-related occupations as recorded in the LFS. The choice of occupations to include is to some extent subjective as many occupations include both care and non-care work. We therefore make judgements about the weight of the care work. For example, we include primary and pre-primary education teaching professionals but exclude secondary and tertiary teachers on the basis that the latter's work will not involve much care.

The calculations yield total earnings of R83,928m, of which R24,128m accrues to male earners and R59,800m to female earners. The most "generous" measure suggests that unpaid care work is equivalent to more than three times the earnings of care workers in the paid economy. The most modest measure also shows unpaid care work having a higher value than these earnings. As before, the extent to which unpaid care work exceeds paid care work is greater for females than for males. The gender gap is smaller than for the earlier comparisons because of the preponderance of women in paid care work. In respect of the narrower person care, the value is nearly 40 per cent of paid care work with the most generous measure, and 15 per cent for the most modest.

CONCLUSION

As so often when analysing care work, there are no big surprises in the overall patterns described before. In particular, the Tobit estimation confirms the expected factors are influencing the amount of care work that women and men, girls and boys do in South Africa. What might be surprising, however, is that marriage is not a significant determinant of the amount of unpaid care work or person care done. Having one's young child living in the same household is, in contrast, a very strong determinant. These findings reflect a society in which many children are born and raised outside of marriage, marriage rates are low, and divorce and separation rates high.

The macro comparisons in the latter part of the paper confirm, by using a range of comparisons, that the amount of unpaid care work and person care done in the economy is huge. Policy-making that ignores something of this size and significance cannot but fail to produce optimal societal outcomes.

Numbers cannot, however, tell us the full story. There might, for example, be factors—such as biases in reporting of person care—that influence some of the patterns. The time use data also cannot tell us much about activities that are done by a relatively small proportion of the population, and or done for relatively short times. The data thus tell us much less about care of elderly and sick adults than they tell us about care of children. These gaps are especially important in a society in the middle of a severe HIV & AIDS pandemic.

REFERENCES

Bakker, Isabella (ed). 1994. *The Strategic Silence*. Zed Books, London.
Budlender, Debbie and Ann Lisbet Brathaug. 2002. *Calculating the Value of Unpaid Labour: A Discussion Document*. Statistics South Africa, Pretoria.
Deaton, Angus. 2003. *Measuring Poverty in a Growing World (or Measuring Growth in a Poor World)*. Working Paper 9822. National Bureau of Economic Research, Cambridge.
National Treasury. 2003a. *Budget Review*. Pretoria.
National Treasury. 2003b. *Intergovernmental Fiscal Review*. Pretoria.

4 Unpaid Care Work
Analysis of the Indian Time Use Data
Neetha N. and Rajni Palriwala

INTRODUCTION

A clear division between paid and unpaid work and between women's care work and economic–work may be possible in countries where fully developed markets have penetrated all sectors of the economy and society. In countries like India, however, it is difficult to make these separations. A large proportion of women constantly move back and forth between care work and "economic" work through the day or these activities are undertaken simultaneously. This is especially the case where women are engaged in "economic" activities for household consumption carried out in the home. These activities are not captured adequately by the labour force data systems. There have been micro-level attempts to document care work and to measure the unpaid work of women—both "economic" and "non-economic". Notwithstanding the efforts of feminist social scientists and activists since the 1970s, it is only in the late 1990s that documentation at the national level was initiated. The Time Use Survey of 1998–1999, which was largely the outcome of these efforts, provided the first opportunity to estimate the time spent on and value of care work and unpaid labour of women in general. Although this was a pilot survey, it continues to be the only time use data for the country.

THE OBJECTIVES AND METHODOLOGY OF THE SURVEY

The Time Use Survey (TUS) was carried out in 1998–1999 by the Central Statistical Organisation (CSO). Unlike the case of some other countries, in India the survey was seen as an instrument for improving statistics on labour and national income, such that estimation of care work was largely secondary. Taking into account the diversity of the country, six states were covered in the survey, covering six different regions of the country and three-staged stratified random sampling was followed for the selection of households. The survey covered 18,591 households, including 77,593 individuals of whom 40,187 were males and 37,406 were females (Central Statistical Organisation 2001).

The survey instrument used was that of interviews on a one-day recall method. The time spent on different activities was to be collected for time slots of one hour each starting from 3.00 a.m in the morning to 24 hours later on the next day, for all days covered by the survey. In the absence of the widespread use of watches and clocks, investigators were trained to collect data chronologically, systematically linking it with other time schedules with which the participants would be familiar (school time, office time, etc.).

Three sets of schedules were used: one for collecting data on characteristics of the selected households, the second on details of individual members of these households, and the third on the time use pattern of all members aged 6 years and above. The time use data were collected for three types of days—normal day, weekly variant day (such as a weekend day) and abnormal day (if such was found)—within a single reference week. The survey was repeated every three months over a period of one year, so as to capture seasonal variations, with different households targeted in each quarter. Information was gathered on simultaneous or multiple activities within each time slot and the total time in any one slot was divided across the various activities on the basis of their relative importance as reported by the informant. However, if economic and non-economic activities were reported simultaneously, the investigators gave priority to economic activities (Government of India 2007). Thus from the very start of the TUS exercise, care work was devalued and likely to be allocated a smaller proportion of the time.

The reported incidence of weekly variant and abnormal days, other than in the state of Meghalaya,[1] was very low as was the seasonal variation. Overall, the normal days constituted 93 per cent of all days covered in the survey and this proportion was marginally higher for women than for men (CSO 2000). Weekly average time spent on various activities was calculated based on the presence of various types of days. In the case of individuals with only normal days, the time spent on various activities on a normal day was multiplied by seven to get the weekly total. In the case of individuals with weekly variant and abnormal days the time spent on a normal day was multiplied by five and the weekly total was calculated by adding an abnormal and the weekly variant day. The weekly total was divided by seven to get the daily average time spent.

A specially designed classification schedule was used for the survey to ensure adequate coverage of activities, as well as compatibility and comparability with other national and international data. The Indian classification did not follow the United Nations Statistics Division (UNSD) (1997) classification which distinguishes between economic categories in terms of whether the work was done in establishments or not. The major classification groups that were used in the time use survey are: primary production activities; secondary production activities; tertiary production activities; household maintenance, management and shopping for own households; care for children, elderly, and disabled of own household; community services; learning; social and cultural activities; personal care and self maintenance. The first three are referred to as System of National Accounts (SNA) activities as they fall within the narrowly defined production boundary; the next three are extended SNA (ESNA), activities which fall within the general production boundary; the last three are non-SNA activities, and do not constitute work. The three groups of activities are further classified at 2-digit and 3-digit levels.

Extended SNA is equivalent to unpaid care work. The 2-digit and 3-digit classifications enables a differentiation between household and extra-household care and, more importantly, between direct and indirect care activities, as will be discussed in subsequent text. Thus, the TUS data allow for an exploration of the differences in care time by household and individual characteristics so as to delineate the factors which influence care patterns at the macro-level.

In the present analysis, all the activities that fall under SNA are referred to as paid work, although there are unpaid components in SNA. The paid activities are considered to be "economic" work and are included in the estimation of gross domestic product. In addition, there are a few components of primary production activities such as processing of products for own consumption which are not included in the estimation of GDP in India, but fall under the SNA category. Further, unlike the standard definitions of employment and unemployment, engagement of persons in SNA work for less than one hour was recorded in the TUS. In addition, travel time for economic work purposes as well as time spent on activities such as fetching water which are not counted in the usual labour force calculations, are included under SNA in the TUS survey. Thus, activities covered under SNA are much broader than the conventional labour force definitions, leading to a difference in labour force estimates of TUS vis-à-vis other sources. Analysis across these broad categories of SNA and extended SNA can give insight into the division between "economic" work and unpaid care work.

All individual data are presented in the following section disaggregated by sex. As mentioned previously, time use data were gathered for individuals aged 6 years and older. Since the data were collected from the respondents themselves, there are likely to be reporting problems with the data from children, especially for those in the younger age categories, although some help was given by parents or caregivers. To circumvent this problem, the disaggregated analysis is limited to individuals aged 10 and older. This is similar to the age group used for time use surveys in many other countries.

TIME ALLOCATION ACROSS UNPAID CARE WORK AND SNA

An overview of respondents (those from whom time use data was collected) in terms of whether they participated only in SNA, only in extended SNA or in both is given in the following table.

Table 4.1 Percentage Distribution of Participants in SNA and Extended SNA Activities

Category		Only SNA	Only ESNA	SNA & ESNA	No SNA or ESNA
Rural	Male	43.8	5.1	40.6	10.5
	Female	2.6	19.1	73.5	4.7
Urban	Male	32.3	9.0	41.7	17.0
	Female	1.7	49.7	41.5	7.1

The gender and urban–rural differences are striking. A large proportion of men did only SNA activities, but this was true for very few women. Most rural women participated in both SNA and unpaid care work, with a much higher participation rate than for men (both rural and urban) and urban women. The largest proportion of urban women engaged in "only extended SNA". The urban–rural comparative of estimates for men, however, is counter-intuitive. In urban areas, where the distinctions between SNA and extended SNA tend to be sharp, the largest proportion of men engaged in both SNA and extended SNA, whereas in rural areas, where SNA and extended SNA can easily flow into each other, the largest grouping of men were reported to be engaged in "only SNA". This possibly reflects specific extended SNA, which in more strictly sex-segregated societies and in urban areas in particular[2] may fall on men rather than women such as shopping and travel related to care of children and elderly. Interestingly, the proportion of men who reported not being involved in either SNA or extended SNA, i.e. they were non-workers, students, care receivers, etc., was more than double the proportion of such women. This is an expected outcome in a highly patriarchal society where boys are more likely to be in school or college, men are more likely to receive care and be allowed leisure, and girls and women are quickly absorbed into care work. Summing up, it may be noted that a large proportion of women were active in both SNA and extended SNA, unlike men, and the female–male difference in SNA was much smaller than that in extended SNA. Thus, gender differentials were sharper in unpaid care work than in "economic" work, such that half the men do not spend any time on unpaid care work, while less than 10 per cent of women fall in this category.

Moving from the mere fact of whether an individual participated in SNA, ESNA or both, the time allocation of individuals across the two broad categories of work—extended SNA and SNA—is given in the following chart. It gives the average daily time in hours spent, which is derived from the weekly totals. In Figure 4.1, the average daily time is calculated in respect of the "actors" i.e. those who actually undertook the activity concerned, and not in respect of the male or female population aged 10 years and older as a whole.

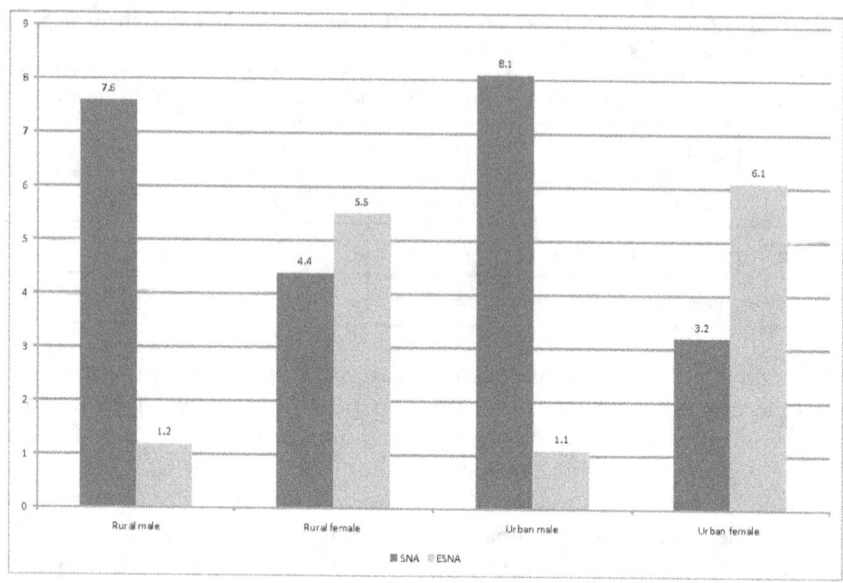

Figure 4.1 Mean hours per day spent by actors on SNA and extended SNA by sex and location.

On average, women spent a significantly larger part of the day in unpaid care work than did men and the male–female differences were very sharp, irrespective of rural/urban location. In rural areas, women who did unpaid care work spent about 5.5 hours of the day on this activity while men who did unpaid care work spent only 1.2 hours of their day on such work. The male–female difference in unpaid care work was slightly larger in urban areas with women spending about 6.1 hours of their day on unpaid care work and men spending more or less the same time as their rural counterparts. Turning to SNA, men who did SNA work on average spent more time on this activity than women, in both rural and urban locations. While for men time spent on SNA was higher in urban areas, for women the reverse was true and the difference was substantial.[3] The longer time spent on SNA by rural women is expected in the context of women's increased contribution in rural agricultural operations.

SOCIO-ECONOMIC VARIABLES AND TIME DISTRIBUTION ACROSS EXTENDED SNA AND SNA

Given the demographic and socio-economic diversity of the country, it is imperative to analyse paid and unpaid work across various socio-economic parameters. Age, marital status, and household size are likely to influence the demand for care and the ability to meet these demands and thence the allocation of time on SNA and ESNA. Caste and religious backgrounds also affect men and women's perceived social roles and responsibilities and thus their time distribution. The employment status of individuals also has a bearing, with the employed having less time to spend on unpaid care work. The role of education on time distribution is much debated due to the mediation of its effects by other social and demographic variables, including entry into employment. For the next set of analyses we report time spent in terms of the population average i.e. calculated across all males or females in the relevant group, whether or not they did SNA or extended SNA. Thus, where the average time is low, it could reflect either a high participation rate with a small amount of time spent by most or a large amount of time spent by a small number of participants. The discussion includes consideration of participation rates, although these are not shown in the figures.

Significant variation is seen across age categories in terms of both SNA and unpaid care work. Women in the peak reproductive age group (18–45) were spending the longest time on care work and had participation rates as high as 98 per cent. For men, the age group 18–45 years reported the highest participation (53 per cent) in rural areas, though the mean time was higher for older, rural men. In urban areas, the 46–64 year age group reported the highest participation (58 per cent) but older men had a higher mean time in care work. This could imply that men participate in unpaid care work once their engagement in SNA declines or ends. In rural areas, the participation rate for SNA for females was found to be highest (84 per cent) in the same age group in which participation in extended SNA was the highest, indicating the extent of a "double burden". Agricultural workers, who work mostly on their own farms, form a large part of this group.

Table 4.2 Mean Hours Spent Daily on SNA and Extended SNA by Age Group

	Age group	Rural		Urban	
		Male	Female	Male	Female
SNA	10–17	4.9	3.3	5.0	2.4
	18–45	8.1	4.5	8.4	3.3
	46–64	7.8	4.8	8.0	3.5
	65+	6.3	3.6	6.4	3.1
ESNA	10–17	1.0	3.0	0.8	2.5
	18–45	1.2	6.4	1.2	7.0
	46–64	1.3	4.7	1.2	5.6
	65+	1.5	4.0	1.5	4.0

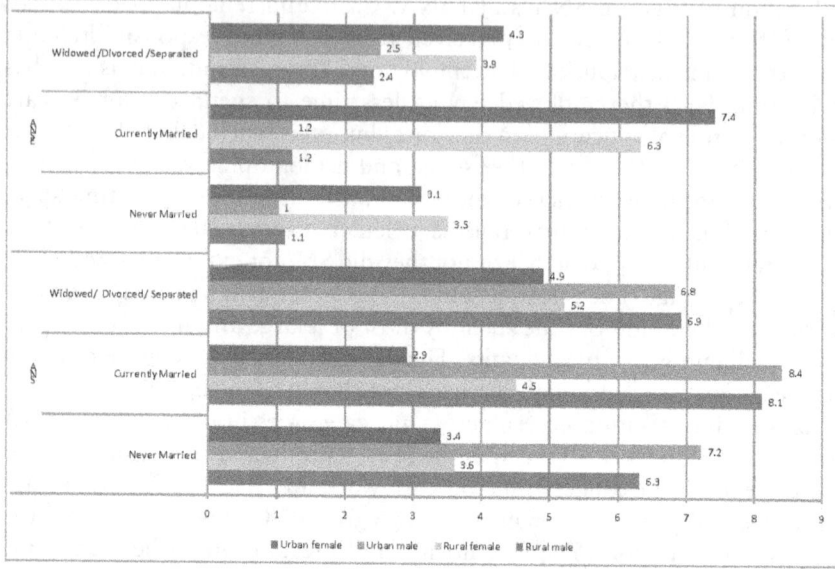

Figure 4.2 Mean hours spent daily on SNA and extended SNA by marital status.

However, in urban areas, while the average time spent on SNA by those in the age group 46–64 was found to be the highest, the participation rate was low across all age categories of women, with those in the age group 18–45 year showing the highest rate, at 49 per cent.

Not only was a higher proportion of widowed, divorced or separated men spending time on care work, they were spending more time on average than the other categories of men across rural and urban areas as shown in Figure 4.2. More striking is the negligible difference in time spent on extended SNA by never married and currently married men. A possible explanation here is that never married men tend to live with other relatives in households in which women are present. Widowed and divorced/separated women spent more time on SNA than other categories of women and their participation rate in unpaid care work was also high. They also spent a substantial amount of time on unpaid care work, only lower than currently married women. This is an expected pattern, in keeping with normative views of the gendered division of labour and local narratives of the particular difficulties which widowed and divorced men and women face.

The time spent on SNA by women showed a negative relationship with the number of members in the household, or in other words, women in households with fewer members spent more time on SNA. However, time spent on unpaid care work increased with the number of members in the households and then showed a decline. This pattern could reflect the household life cycle. As households expand through births and marriages, the demand for care work increases, while the eldest generation contains both members who are active in care work and those who require help. In the course of time, although the number of members may have further increased, older children not only require less care labour from others, but they may also share the burden of care work. Women in households with 3–4 members spent the most time on unpaid care work across rural and urban areas. In contrast to women, the time men spent on unpaid care work showed a decline with increase in household size for both rural and urban areas, confirming the release of male members from unpaid care work with the increase in the number of women in the households. However, the participation rate was highest for women and men with smaller households (1–2). Respectively 97 per cent and 96 per cent of all women and 59 per cent and 66 per cent of all men in rural areas and urban areas reported participating in ESNA.

The first category in Table 4.3, "child 0–6", denotes individuals with children only in the age group of 0–6 in their households. The second category, "child 0–14" may have children in the age category of 0–6 but also have at least one child in the age group of 7–14. Likewise, "child 0–17" may have children in the age group of 0–6 and 7–14 but also have at least a child in the age group of 15–17. Accordingly, the data reveals that, in rural as well as in urban areas, women with only young children in their household spent more time on extended SNA compared to women with both younger and older children. Not only does the demand for care reduce as children get older, the latter can help in caring for younger siblings or in other care work. Furthermore, women with no children younger than the

Table 4.3 Mean Hours Spent Daily on Extended SNA and SNA for Individuals with Children in Their Households

	Age of child/children	Rural		Urban	
		Male	Female	Male	Female
SNA	Child 0–6	7.9	4.2	8.3	2.9
	Child 0–14	7.6	4.2	8.2	3.0
	Child 0–17	7.6	4.3	8.1	3.0
	No children	7.7	4.8	8.0	3.8
ESNA	Child 0–6	1.2	6.2	1.2	7.1
	Child 0–14	1.2	5.8	1.1	6.4
	Child 0–17	1.2	5.7	1.1	6.3
	No children	1.3	5.1	1.3	5.5

age of 18 spent the least time on extended SNA, indicating the importance of childcare in care activity. In contrast, the time spent by men on extended SNA hardly varied with the age of children in the household and was the highest in households with no children. This means that in the absence of children, who may contribute substantially to household work, men tend to spend more time on unpaid care work. The reverse of this pattern is evident with SNA. The time spent by men declines slightly with age of children and the absence of children, suggesting a link between SNA for men and the responsibility of supporting children. Women with younger children spent less time on SNA than all other categories of respondents. Those with no children spent the most time in comparison with their female peers, pointing to the inverse relation between childcare responsibility and labour market participation.

There was no clear variation in time spent on SNA or unpaid care work by women across various religions. On the whole, Hindu women spent more time on SNA in rural and urban areas compared to Muslim women, which is in line with the stereotype of secluded, "non-working" Muslim woman. Urban Hindu women also spent more time on unpaid care work than women of other religions. This may be due to the factors discussed previously—care tasks which require presence in public places and differences in religious restrictions placed on women's presence and mobility outside the home.

The male–female difference in time spent on extended SNA and SNA is significant across key social groupings. In both urban and rural locations, Scheduled Caste (SC) and Scheduled Tribe (ST) women spent more time than other women on SNA. This is in keeping with social science findings and common wisdom about the comparative, gendered patterns in paid work among different social groups in India and with the lower economic standing of SC/ST households compared to others which drives all members into SNA work. The reverse pattern was the case in respect of unpaid care work, though the difference was smaller. For men, there was no difference in time spent on extended SNA between the two social groupings in rural areas, but in urban areas SC/ST category spent more time on extended SNA than other men.

Turning to education, income and employment status, the data shows that in rural areas the amount of time spent on SNA is the highest for men and women who are either illiterate or have less than primary level of education.

The urban figures do not follow the same pattern. The time spent on extended SNA does not seem to have any correlation with education level for the six areas combined. The participation rate, however, reveals interesting patterns. The participation rate is highest for the educational category graduate and above for both men and women across rural and urban areas. While the numbers of graduates is relatively low, this pattern contrasts with the image of the "illiterate housewife".

Table 4.4 Mean Hours Spent Daily on SNA and Unpaid Care Work by Educational Status

	Level of education	Rural		Urban	
		Male	Female	Male	Female
SNA	Illiterate and below primary	7.9	4.8	8.3	3.9
	Primary to higher secondary	7.4	3.4	8.2	2.6
	Graduate and above	6.6	3.7	7.5	4.1
ESNA	Illiterate and below primary	1.2	5.5	1.4	6.2
	Illiterate and below primary	1.2	5.5	1.1	6.1
	Graduate and above	1.4	5.6	1.1	5.8

Households are classified in respect of monthly per capita household expenditures[4] into three broad categories representing those with low, middle and high expenditures. To take into account rural-urban differences in income and monetisation, different expenditure categories have been used for rural and urban areas. In rural areas, the "low" category includes per capita expenditure groups Rs. 0–400, while in urban areas it includes Rs. 0–700. Middle or medium expenditure in rural areas comprise those in the expenditure classes Rs. 401–800 and in urban areas those in the expenditure group Rs. 701–1400. Expenditure categories above Rs. 800 are classified as high in rural areas, while in urban areas this category consists of those individuals with household expenditure above Rs. 1400.

Women in the lower expenditure classes spent more of their daily time on SNA, both in rural and urban areas. While women in the upper expenditure bracket spent only 4.1 hours per day on SNA in rural areas, the time spent was 4.5 hours for the lowest expenditure category. It is, thus, not the failure to work that can explain their poverty. In urban areas the time spent increased for the highest expenditure category after a decline for the middle-income group, which reflects the tendency of the middle class households to comply with respectability norms of "non-working" women. In the case of extended SNA, the time spent by higher expenditure classes was marginally higher than that of lower expenditure classes in rural areas,

Table 4.5 Mean Hours Spent Daily on SNA and Unpaid Care Work by Monthly Per Capita Expenditure

	Expenditure category	Rural		Urban	
		Male	Female	Male	Female
SNA	Low	7.7	4.5	8.2	3.7
	Middle	7.6	4.3	8.0	2.9
	High	7.5	4.1	7.6	3.4
ESNA	Low	1.2	5.5	1.2	6.0
	Middle	1.2	5.6	1.1	6.1
	High	1.3	5.7	1.1	5.9

possibly due to embellishments in household maintenance and the consequent expansion of domestic work in better-off households. However, the urban picture differed with households in the upper middle expenditure groups reporting less time spent on extended SNA. This could be because of the hiring of domestic workers by urban, higher income households, relieving women in the household from this work.

In India, the term "organised sector" is almost identical to the concept of "formal sector" in most other countries. Similarly, the "unorganised sector" is more or less equivalent to the informal sector. Not much difference was found between men in these two sectors in respect of the time spent on unpaid care work. The participation rate, however, differed considerably with a higher rate for men in the organised sector, which was not in keeping with representations of the gender division of labour in this sector. Women in the unorganised sector spent a larger share of their day on unpaid care work than their counterparts in the organised sector with a small variation in participation rates. A considerable proportion of women

Table 4.6 Mean Hours Spent Daily on SNA and Unpaid Care Work by Workers in Organised and Unorganised Sector

	Sector	Rural		Urban	
		Male	Female	Male	Female
SNA	Organised	7.9	6.4	7.9	6.2
	Unorganised	8.2	6.1	8.7	6.1
ESNA	Organised	1.2	4.3	1.2	4.2
	Unorganised	1.2	4.9	1.0	4.8

workers in the unorganised sector are home-based workers, who would normally be combining unpaid care work with SNA. That male workers in the unorganised sector spent more time in SNA than did those in the organised sector is an expected pattern, given the long working hours and the virtual absence of any regulation in the former sector. However, what is interesting is the reverse pattern among women. This could be attributed to the increased proportion of subsidiary workers[5] among women, who may spend much fewer hours in such economic activity.

The survey also collected information from respondents on their usual principal activity status using subcategories utilised in the standard Employment and Unemployment survey. The definition of economic activity is very limited and the data give only the main status of the respondents. However, this classification does help to disaggregate data across paid and unpaid categories of labour. It can also be used to differentiate those outside the workforce into those who engage mainly in housework and others.

Focussing on the presence or absence of monetary income, the various subcategories are grouped into four categories in Table 4.7. Remunerated occupations includes employers, paid home-based workers, permanent and non-permanent employees, casual and contractual wage labourers in public and other works, paid trainees, and beggars and commercial sex workers. Unremunerated occupations include unpaid helpers in household enterprises, exchange labourers, and those doing domestic duties while also engaged in unpaid collection of goods, sewing, tailoring, weaving etc., for household use. Housework covers those doing unpaid domestic duties in their own household, while the fourth category covers the unemployed, full-time students, pensioners, and those unable to work.

Table 4.7 shows that even if we exclude those who were only engaged in unpaid household duties (i.e. who did unpaid care work), men and women engaged in unremunerated occupations spent more time on unpaid care

Table 4.7 Mean Hours Spent Daily on Extended SNA Across Activity Classification Groups

	Rural		Urban	
	Male	Female	Male	Female
Remunerated occupations	1.2	4.5	1.1	4.5
Unremunerated occupations	1.3	5.6	1.4	6.2
Housework	3.7	7.0	4.3	7.4
Others/Out of the workforce	1.1	2.6	1.2	2.5

work than those engaged in paid work. The difference between the two was particularly marked for women. Thus, the very fact of being in unremunerated rather than paid work seems to place a greater burden of unpaid care work on them, while paid labour excused workers from care work.

The aforementioned analysis is based on the average time spent on unpaid care work calculated across the full male/female group, whether or not particular individuals engaged in the activity. As indicated earlier, the average value is affected by the number of individuals doing the activity, i.e. the participation rate. Thus, the average value can have a low value even if some individuals spent considerable time on unpaid care work. Since gender appears as the most important differentiator of time spent in various activities, to get an idea on the dispersion of the actual time and the number of individuals spending longer or shorter hours, men and women were classified across time slots of half an hour using the full minute daily time spent on unpaid care work (UCW).

The distribution of UCW is asymmetric for both male and female. These are clearly not normal distributions, but the distribution for women has an extremely long tail, while the distribution for men has a short tail. The short tail for males suggests a low variability, i.e. males do a fairly consistently low amount of UCW. The long tail for women suggests the opposite—high variability and differences among women.

Men were concentrated in the time slots of less than one hour with very few men reporting more than two and a half hours of unpaid care work. Women too were concentrated in the lower time slots. However, a

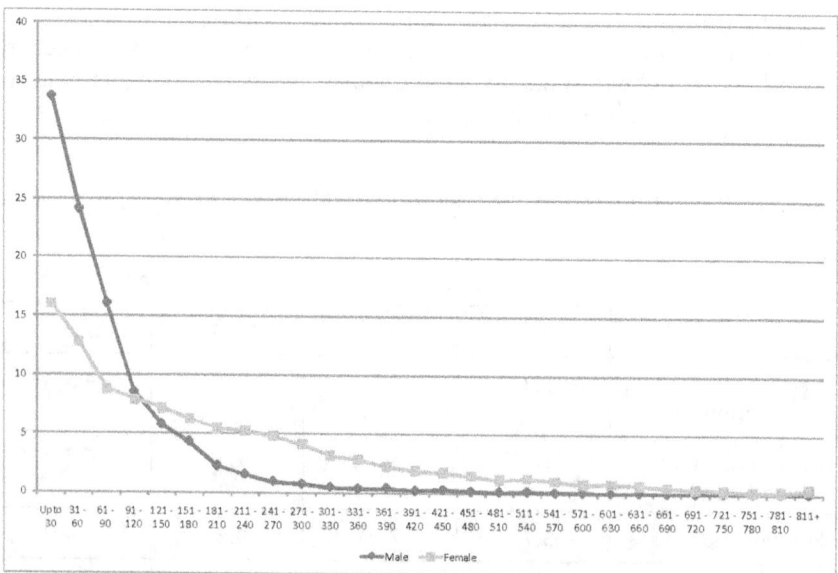

Figure 4.3 Distribution of number of persons across various time slots spent on unpaid care work.

substantial number of women were seen in the upper time slots and they were more evenly spread across various time categories. At one end of the scale, close to 35 per cent of males and 15 per cent of females spent no time on unpaid care work on any average day. At the other end, a large number of women spent 8, or more than 8 hours while not even a single man did so.

COMPONENTS OF UNPAID CARE WORK

As noted earlier, unpaid care work consists of a varied number of activities, which were broadly classified into three categories in the survey: household maintenance, management and shopping for own household; care for children, sick, elderly and disabled for own household; and community services and help to other households. In this section, a disaggregation across these broad activities as well as subcategories within them is undertaken so as to unbundle care work. Of these categories, the second, care for children, sick, elderly and disabled of own household is referred to as "person care" (or care of persons) in all the subsequent discussions.

Table 4.8 gives the average daily time spent on the three broad categories of extended SNA or unpaid care work, for males and females as well as across rural and urban areas.

Women spent more time than men on all categories of unpaid care work. Rural men spent more time on unpaid care work compared to urban men, the reverse being true for women. Of all the unpaid care work categories, men spent the maximum proportion of time on community services and help to other households in rural areas. This was not the case in urban areas.

Women spent by far the maximum part of their unpaid care time on household maintenance and shopping for own household. Although there was a large difference in time spent by men and women on person care, the difference was much sharper in the case of household maintenance. The low amount of time spent on person care could be because some part of

Table 4.8 Mean Hours Spent Daily on Subcategories of Unpaid Care Work

	Rural		Urban		Total	
	Male	Female	Male	Female	Male	Female
Household maintenance	1.0	4.9	1.0	5.3	1.0	5.0
Person care	1.0	1.7	0.9	1.9	0.9	1.8
Community service	1.2	1.3	1.0	1.1	1.1	1.2

such work was carried out simultaneously with cooking and other household work and even alongside paid work, especially home-based work. In a 24-hour calculation of average daily time, if multiple activities are performed by an individual simultaneously, the time spent on each activity gets reduced. Furthermore, as discussed before, in such situations the TUS gave priority to "economic activity" in dividing the time recorded for each.

To capture unpaid care time taking into account simultaneity, the full minute measure was calculated using the data on simultaneous activities.

With the full minute calculation we get higher values for all categories of unpaid care work than with the 24-hour calculation, showing the prevalence of simultaneity in care work. However, the difference is small which suggests the possibility of underreporting and misreporting of multiple activities.

CARE OF CHILDREN, THE SICK, ELDERLY AND DISABLED HOUSEHOLD MEMBERS

Person care is the category which assumes significance in most contemporary discussions on care work. It constitutes the second largest category within unpaid care work in terms of time allocation by individuals, but even then adds up to a small part of the day. Within this category of care, childcare and adult care were recorded separately in the Indian TUS, and hence one can analyse the pattern across these categories. Before focussing on childcare, the picture for the care of the sick, elderly and disabled household members in rural and urban areas is discussed.

Care for adults in the household is captured under three sub-categories in the survey: physical care of the sick, disabled, elderly household members: washing, dressing, feeding, helping;[6] supervising adults needing care—with or without other activities; and travel related to the care of adults and others. Only 382 men and 1,206 females were found to participate in this care work of the total surveyed at the all India level, of which 231 men and 868 women were from rural areas and the remainder (151 males and 338 females) were from urban areas.

The gender difference in person care for adults is very small in absolute terms and also in relative terms for rural people and overall. However women clearly invested more time than men. The participation rate is also

Table 4.9 Mean Hours Spent Daily on Care for Sick, Disabled and Elderly

Rural		Urban		Total	
Male	Female	Male	Female	Male	Female
1.0	1.1	0.7	1.2	0.9	1.1

extremely low. To some extent this could be due to underreporting of such work. However, this also points to the absence of special care arrangements for the old, the sick and the disabled at the household level in the country, despite the rhetoric that the Indian family takes care of its old and sick.

As noted earlier, within the category of care for children, the sick, elderly and disabled of own household, there are specific codes which record time spent on childcare work. These are: 511—physical care of children, washing, dressing, feeding; 521—teaching training and instruction to own children; 531—accompanying children to places: school, sports, lessons etc, primary health care (PHC), doctor; 561—supervising children needing care; and 571—travel related to care of children. In the following analysis, these sub-categories are defined as direct childcare as care for children in its broader sense should also take into account time spent on household tasks such as cooking and cleaning, without which childcare cannot take place. In Table 4.10 time spent by men and women who engage in these activities (grouped together) are given.

The gender difference in direct childcare was much sharper than that in adult care, with women spending more than double the time on childcare than men did. While the average daily time spent by women on direct childcare was higher than that spent on adult care, it remained extremely low. This could be attributed to the simultaneity that exists between other work and childcare work, especially childminding. The last can be low intensity, but long duration work. As noted previously, the Indian methodology explicitly prioritised SNA when simultaneous SNA work and unpaid care work were reported. Within this, it would appear that child-minding and supervision are particularly devalued, both in terms of recognition and in terms of time spent on it if it occurs at the same time as other activities.

Although direct childcare occupies such a small part of the day for women and men, its variation along various individual and household characteristics is examined, in the hope that this very issue (the little time spent on it) may be further illuminated. Accordingly in the following section, average daily time spent by men and women on direct childcare is disaggregated by various demographic and socio-economic variables.

Women in the older age groups, especially 65+ spent more time on direct childcare than all others. Girls in the age group 10–17 and men aged 65 years and more spent the same average time on childcare, only a little less than women in the age group 18–44. Boys in the age group 10–17 also

Table 4.10 Mean Daily Hours Spent on Direct Child Care Activities

Rural		Urban		Total	
Male	Female	Male	Female	Male	Female
1.2	3.1	1.1	3.9	1.2	3.3

Table 4.11 Time Spent and Participation in Direct Chid Care by Demographic and Social Variables

Variables	Categories	Male		Female	
		Hours	Participation rate	Hours	Participation rate
Age groups	10–17	1.1	5.1	1.3	14.2
	18–45	0.8	21.1	1.4	60.6
	46–64	0.9	10.8	1.7	29.1
	65+	1.3	11.6	2.1	23.0
Marital status	Never married	0.9	4.6	1.3	13.9
	Currently married	0.8	22.2	1.4	60.3
	Widowed/Divorced/Separated	1.3	15.1	1.7	27.2
Household size	1–2	0.6	6.1	1.0	11.3
	3–4	0.9	17.4	1.7	40.4
	5–6	1.0	16.4	1.8	42.2
	6	0.8	16.7	1.9	51.1
Age of children	0–6	1.0	27.8	2.0	67.2
	0–14	1.0	20.8	1.9	51.7
	0–17	1.0	18.9	1.8	47.7
	No children	0.6	6.0	1.0	12.9
Caste groups	SC/ST	1.0	16.9	1.7	42.5
	Others	0.9	15.3	1.8	38.8

spent only a little less time than their female peers.[7] Thus, although the eldest women and women in the reproductive ages are the most involved in childcare, the last is shared across the household, with siblings and grandparents pitching in. Fathers and men in the work force, however, do the least of such work.

Widowed, divorced or separated women spent more daily time on childcare work, although they were less likely to participate in this work than currently married women. Widowed, divorced or separated men spent more daily time on childcare than other men. Clearly, with the absence of a partner, this (and other direct care work) fell on these men. This is especially so for widowed men, because children of divorced or separated men often live with their mothers. Strikingly, men who were never married spent a larger part of their day on childcare than did currently married men, which is congruent with the time use pattern by age. Thus, brothers and uncles are more likely to look after children than are fathers, a pattern noted in ethnographic studies.

Time spent on direct childcare by women increases with household size, most sharply in the move from households consisting of only 1–2 members to those of 3–4 members, i.e. from households in which there would be one child at the most to those in which there could be any number from 1–3. This higher average value for larger households could be partly attributed to the presence of more children. Further, many smaller households may have only older people, as their children might have left them and are living separately, reducing the time spent on childcare by members of these households. With men, in contrast, the average daily time spent on direct childcare decreases in the largest size category of households, perhaps because older children-siblings take over from parents.

As expected, the time spent on direct childcare declined with the presence of older children, for both men and women. The surprise is that members of households with no children younger than 18 years of age spent time on direct childcare, though it was much less than for households with resident children. This indicates the possibility of day care of children of neighbours or kin.

A comparison across religious categories shows no clear pattern, except that women in the "others" category spent less time than Hindus or Muslims. SC women spent less time on direct childcare than others, though the difference was very small. The reverse was the case for men. This could be on account of the lower socio-economic status of SCs and STs in general compared to other social categories, leading to the greater engagement of women in non-household paid work and/or the greater simultaneity among them of paid work and care work as well as the irregularity of employment for SC/ST men.

Much of the discussion in India on childcare has revolved around the idea that illness and mortality among children is a result of uneducated women not giving "proper" care to their children. It is presumed that it is education and knowledge which are lacking rather than the means for care. Although time spent is not a direct indication of the quality of care, illiterate and below primary educated women spent more time compared to other categories. The pattern was similar with illiterate and less educated men spending more time on childcare compared to other categories.

Women in the middle expenditure category spent the most time on childcare work, while the high income category reported the least time. In terms of participation, however, the lowest income group recorded the maximum

Table 4.12 Time Spent and Participation in Direct Chid Care by Education and Economic Variables

Variables	Categories	Male		Female	
		Hours	Participation rate	Hours	Participation rate
Education	Illiterate and below primary	0.9	11.8	1.5	40.4
	Primary to higher secondary	0.8	19.9	1.4	48.5
	Graduate and above	0.8	4.7	1.2	6.2
Expenditure	Low	1.0	15.8	1.7	42.3
	Medium	0.9	15.9	1.8	38.2
	High	0.9	15.2	1.5	29.9
Sectors	Organised	0.8	31.2	0.9	46.5
	Unorganised	0.7	51.8	1.1	42.4
Work Status	Remunerated occupations	0.9	4.1	1.3	40.9
	Unremunerated occupations	0.9	6.2	1.6	50.4
	Housework	1.0	17.1	1.7	65.6
	Others	1.9	0.9	2.0	24.4

rate, with the rate dropping as expenditure increased. As noted earlier, this may be the outcome of norms of the non-working mother/wife and the employment of maids/nannies among the middle and higher income categories on the one hand and the necessity for poor women to combine non-household paid work with care activities on the other. It could also reflect higher rates of childbearing among lower-income groups. For men the time spent hardly varied with expenditure category.

Women working in the unorganised sector reported relatively more time spent on direct childcare. For men, the pattern was reversed, and those working in the organised sector spent more time on direct childcare work than their counterparts in the unorganised sector. Unpaid workers, both men and women, spent a larger share of their day on childcare than did

Table 4.13 Mean Daily Hours Spent on Subcategories of Direct Child Care

	Rural		Urban		Total	
	Male	Female	Male	Female	Male	Female
Physical care of children	1.0	2.1	0.8	2.4	0.9	2.2
Teaching, training, etc.	1.2	1.3	1.0	1.7	1.1	1.5
Accompanying children to places	1.1	1.1	0.5	0.9	0.8	1.0
Supervising children	1.1	2.8	1.0	2.6	1.1	2.8
Travel related to care of children	0.4	0.7	0.3	0.7	0.4	0.7

paid workers. For women, of all the categories of usual status activities it was the category "others" who spent the most time on care work, even more than women who reported "housework" as their usual status.

The aforementioned analysis of direct childcare groups together various activities of childcare. Disaggregation of the latter may give further insights into the gendered nature of time spent on specific tasks of direct childcare.

Both rural and urban women spent substantially more time than men on physical care of children and on supervising children. Women also spent more of their time than did men on teaching, training and instruction of own child, particularly in urban areas. Given the female–male literacy gap, especially in rural India, this would be surprising, unless we view it as another indication of the strong gendering of childcare. In the category travel related to the care of children, though women spent more time than men, the gender difference was not as pronounced as for physical care and supervision. A complete reversal of the gender pattern was observed for the category "accompanying children to places" in rural areas. The pattern in these two categories of care activity is in keeping with the point made earlier regarding restrictions on women's mobility in public places and dealings.

As with the broader categories of activities, the distribution of time spent by men and women in person care (all categories together) was plotted across various time slots, showing the dispersion pattern. The graph is very similar to the earlier one: a concentration in the shorter duration slots and the number of women and men declining as duration increases; and a more even distribution of women compared to men across the duration spectrum.

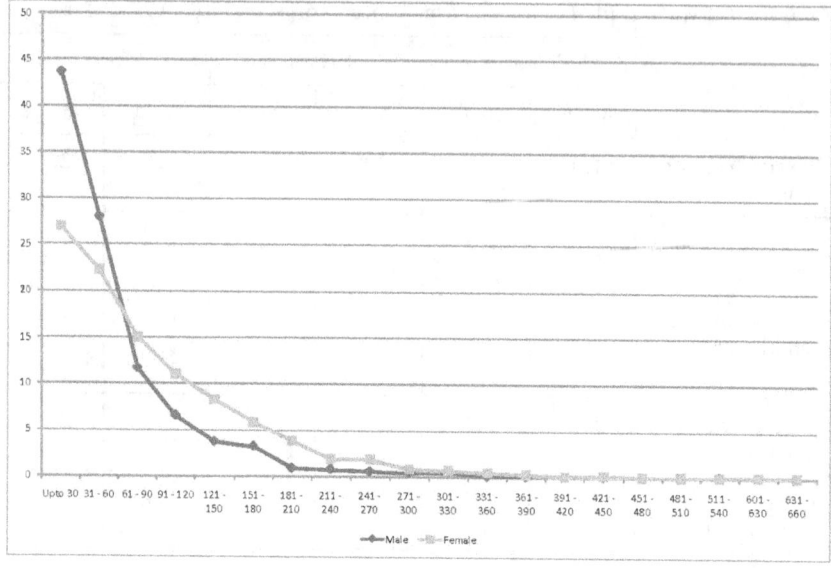

Figure 4.4 Distribution of population by sex and time spent on person care.

A substantial number of women are found in all the time slots of less than 4 hours. At one end of the scale, close to 45 per cent of males and 30 per cent of females spent no time on childcare work on an average day. At the other end, very few men spent more than 4 hours, while more than 2 per cent of women spent longer than 5 hours on childcare work.

HOUSEHOLD MAINTENANCE AND SHOPPING FOR OWN HOUSEHOLD

As is evident from the data on the disaggregated categories of unpaid care work, one of the most important components of care work is the time spent on household maintenance and related work. As discussed earlier, care for children in its wider sense must take into account the time spent not only on direct attendance and care of children, but also that spent on tasks such as cooking food for them or cleaning their immediate environment, without which childcare cannot take place. The importance of this supportive work is evident from the patterns of time spent by both men and women across households with children of different ages, although we cannot distinguish the household maintenance that supports childcare from other household maintenance.

Table 4.14 shows that average daily time spent on household maintenance by women declined with an increase in the age of children in the household for both rural and urban areas. What is striking, however, is the large proportion of time spent on household maintenance by individuals

Table 4.14 Time Spent and Participation in Household Maintenance by the Presence of Children in Different Age Categories

Age categories of children	Male		Female	
	Hours	Participation rate	Hours	Participation rate
0–6	0.9	42.3	5.2	90.9
0–14	0.9	40.3	5.0	89.3
0–17	0.9	39.8	5.0	89.5
None	1.3	46.2	5.1	93.9

who did not report the presence of children younger than 18 years of age in their household. In households without children, while younger children requiring more unpaid care work may be absent, also absent are older children who could share household maintenance tasks. The relatively large amount could also be attributed to the relative absence of multi-tasking in households without children due to childcare not being required, such that the time spent on household maintenance gets captured in full. In contrast, in households with children in which individuals carry out household maintenance work alongside childcare, the total time is divided across these activities, which would give lower figures for all the activities concerned.

COMMUNITY SERVICES

In the third category of extended SNA, community services and help to other households, some categories prima facie have little or no bearing on person care, especially childcare. Hence, these categories were excluded from our detailed analysis. However, we give a brief picture of a few categories, grouped together, which could be taken as having some connection with childcare. The activities are volunteering with/for an organisation (which does not involve working directly for individuals); volunteer work through organisations extended directly to individuals and groups; and informal help to other households.

Table 4.15 Mean Daily Hours Spent on Childcare-related Community Services and Help to Other Households

Rural		Urban		Total	
Male	Female	Male	Female	Male	Female
1.2	2.9	1.1	1.8	1.2	2.5

Gender differences clearly existed in the case of time spent on these community services, and rural women spent a larger share of their day on community services compared to urban women. Thus in almost all categories of extended SNA, and especially those related to childcare, the pattern was clearly one of where women spent more time. Further, both the participation rate and the time spent tended to be greater for women who had younger children, smaller household size (thus less help within the household), and who were not in paid work. However, even women in paid work spent more time than men in their households.

KEY DETERMINANTS OF TIME SPENT ON UNPAID CARE WORK

The previous analysis revealed the influence of multiple socio-economic variables on the likelihood of participation and quantum of time spent on care work. To test the relative strength of relationships between these variables and time spent on care, a Tobit regression model was used. Two Tobit estimations are done: one for unpaid care work as a whole, and the second for person care. Since community care, i.e. time spent on care of persons in other households was negligible, it was not included in the estimation of person care.

Table 4.16 Tobit Regression Results for Time Spent on Unpaid Care Work

	Coef.	Std. Err.	t	P>t	95% Conf. Interval	
Male	-5.136	0.029	-176.070	0.000	-5.193	-5.079
SC	-0.116	0.034	-3.420	0.001	-0.182	-0.050
Married	1.950	0.034	56.910	0.000	1.883	2.017
Rural	-0.103	0.029	-3.520	0.000	-0.161	-0.046
Illiterate	0.071	0.029	2.430	0.015	0.014	0.128
Employed	-1.555	0.030	-50.980	0.000	-1.615	-1.495
Children <18	0.154	0.033	4.610	0.000	0.088	0.219
Age	0.226	0.005	49.800	0.000	0.218	0.235
Age squared	-0.003	0.000	-54.590	0.000	-0.003	-0.003
HH Exp	0.000	0.000	-1.890	0.059	0.000	0.000
Hh size	-0.077	0.007	-10.600	0.000	-0.091	-0.062
Constant	1.250	0.081	15.430	0.000	1.092	1.409

The dependent variable is the time spent on unpaid care work. The explanatory variables include both continuous and discrete/dummy variables. Age, age squared, monthly household expenditure and household size are the continuous variables. The selected dummy variables are: Male, SC (scheduled caste), Married, Illiterate, Employed, Rural, and Children <18 (presence of a child in the household). The result from the Tobit estimation is given in 0.

The results confirm that all the factors except household monthly expenditure and educational attainment are significant (p<0.05) determinants of time spent on unpaid care work. The results indicate higher values of time spent on unpaid care work for those who are female, currently married, urban, and have children younger than the age of 18 years. In contrast, time spent on unpaid care work tends to be less for the Scheduled Castes and among the employed. Time spent on unpaid care work, as expected, tends to increase with age. However, age squared showed a decline indicating a decrease in time spent on unpaid care work among the oldest age groups. Finally, there tends to be a decline in time spent on unpaid care work with increase in household size.

For the second estimation time spent on person care is the dependent variable while the explanatory variables are the same as in the case of unpaid care work.

Table 4.17 Tobit Regression Results for Time Spent on Person Care

	Coef.	Std. Err.	t	P>t	95% Conf. Interval	
Male	-1.555	0.030	-52.030	0.000	-5.193	-5.079
SC	-0.015	0.033	-0.460	0.001	-0.182	-0.050
Married	1.713	0.037	46.360	0.000	1.883	2.017
Rural	-0.296	0.028	-10.420	0.000	-0.161	-0.046
Illiterate	0.059	0.028	2.120	0.015	0.014	0.128
Employed	-0.450	0.030	-15.170	0.000	-1.615	-1.495
Children <18	1.943	0.039	49.390	0.000	0.088	0.219
Age	0.020	0.004	4.400	0.000	0.218	0.235
Age squared	-0.000	0.000	-5.210	0.000	-0.003	-0.003
HH Exp	0.000	0.000	-2.660	0.059	0.000	0.000
Hh size	0.047	0.007	7.050	0.000	-0.091	-0.062
Constant	-3.376	0.084	-40.260	0.000	1.092	1.409

The results shows that all the factors except caste are significant ($p<0.05$) determinants of time spent on person care. As in the case of unpaid care work as a whole, females, urban people, those currently married, and those in households with children younger than age 18 years tend to spend more time on person care, while the employed spend less time. Education is also found to be significant with illiterate people spending more time on person care. In the case of age and age squared the relation was found to be the same as in the case of unpaid care work. Monthly expenditure and household size show a positive relation indicating an increase in time spent on person care with increase in monthly expenditure and household size.

CONCLUSION

The analysis of various dimensions of care work, time allocation patterns and their relationship to various socio-economic characteristics of care givers provided the broader picture within which care work takes place at the household level. The structure of the household in terms of size, presence and age of children, and urban-rural location affect the demand for care, while the gender, economic and other personal characteristics of the individual influence how much time they spend on unpaid care work. The effects of caste or religious group on time spent on care are not direct, but are possibly mediated by other factors such as occupation, economic resources and location.

We have also gained some insight into the labour-care regimes. Thus, participation in unpaid care work and participation in paid work are correlated. The market—the availability of care givers and the need for livelihoods—affects the relations and extent of care work in the household. Yet women who spent time in paid work also spent more time than men in unpaid care work. It is not possible from the numbers to say whether the first determines the second or vice versa and whether causation works in the same way for men and women. The data made available to us through the TUS also carry biases in reporting and non-reporting of care time. Further, it has not been possible to delineate the impact of non-household carers, individual, community or institutional, on the time use patterns of individuals at the household level. These dimensions and theirs complexities are issues that the survey does not address.

NOTES

1. Meghalaya has a large proportion of Christians who observe Sunday as a compulsory break from work.
2. In many parts of India, many women do not go, or at least do not go unaccompanied, to public places such as markets, hospitals, schools or places where they will have to deal with men who are "strangers". In urban areas, not only

is the location of these public places more clearly demarcated from residences, but men may undertake the necessary tasks while commuting to work.
3. The difference is also captured by other data sources.
4. In India, rather than income figures, monthly per capita expenditure data are collected in most national level surveys.
5. Subsidiary workers are workers who pursue activities other than "economic activities" during a major part of the reference year. Thus they denote workers who do some "economic" work during the year, but for short duration, and are unemployed or non-workers in terms of principal status.
6. Within this category, the disabled could possibly include children. However, given the low numbers we have here and the clear separation of other childcare, we have included this sub-category with the care of adults.
7. The small sample size among age group 65+ could affect the reliability of these results.

REFERENCES

Central Statistical Organisation. 2001. *Applications of Time Use Statistics 2001.* Proceedings of the National Seminar on Applications of Time Use Statistics, 8–19 October. Central Statistical Organisation, New Delhi.

Central Statistical Organisation. 2000. *Report of the Time Use Survey.* Ministry of Statistics and Programme Implementation, New Delhi.

Government of India. 2007. *Towards Mainstreaming Time Use Surveys in National Statistical System in India.* Proceedings of the International Seminar on Towards Mainstreaming Time Use Surveys in National Statistical System in India, 24–25 May, Goa. Ministry of Women and Child Development, New Delhi.

5 Republic of Korea
Analysis of Time Use Survey on Work and Care

Mi-young An

INTRODUCTION

This chapter analyses time use data to explore work and care regimes in the Republic of Korea (Korea hereafter). The National Statistics Office (NSO) has conducted time use surveys (TUS) every five years from 1999, with the aim of collecting information on how people spend their time during a 24-hour period. Through the analysis of time use data, this chapter aims firstly to analyse how individuals from different socio-economic backgrounds and different types of households allocate their time to paid and unpaid care work. Secondly, it aims to compare the monetary value of unpaid care work with various macro-economic indicators.

The instrument for the 1999 TUS consists of two parts: the household characteristics questionnaire and the time-diary schedule. The first part collected data on household characteristics, including composition of the household, nature of dwelling, car ownership, and care for preschool children. It also collected information on individual characteristics of household members including gender, age, education, marital status, employment status, occupation, weekly working time, status of workers and subjective evaluation of time pressure and tiredness. In the 2004 survey, the household and individual questionnaires were separated and the instrument thus includes three parts: the household questionnaire, the individual questionnaire for respondents 10 years of age and older, and the time-diary. In both surveys, all the household members aged 10 and older were asked to record their main and simultaneous activities in the time diary, which was structured in 10-minute slots for the designated two days.

The 1999 survey sample was generated from the multi-purpose household sample which was derived from the 1995 population and housing census, using three-stage stratified sampling methods. The 1999 sample consists of 42,953 individuals aged 10 and older and 16,389 households from 850 enumerator districts. The 2004 TUS sample also was generated from the multipurpose household sample, which this time was derived from the 2000 population and housing census, using three-stage stratified sampling methods. The 2004 sample consists of 31,634 individuals aged 10 years and older and 12,651 households from 850 enumerator districts. The data from both surveys were subsequently weighted to be representative of the population aged 10 years above of the country as a whole.

All the self-recorded activities in the time diary, in both the 1999 and 2004 data, are post-coded to three-digit codes, which are divided into nine broad categories. The nine categories are:

1) personal care activities
2) employment
3) study
4) household maintenance
5) family care
6) voluntary service
7) leisure
8) travel
9) others

Personal care comprises activities such as sleeping, eating and drinking, personal hygiene and health care. Household maintenance comprises activities such as food preparation, clothes care, cleaning, purchasing goods for household care, and so forth. Family care comprises activities such as care for family members including infants, children, spouses, parents and other family members. Voluntary service comprises helping neighbours and volunteer activities. The 1999 data are coded according to 137 activity categories, and the 2004 data according to 125 activity categories. The changes in codes between 1999 and 2004 included some that relate to paid work and unpaid care work and which thus affect our analysis.

DESCRIPTION OF 1999 AND 2004 TUS

This section describes the 1999 and 2004 TUS. The focus of the research is on gender differences, thus all the outcomes are disaggregated by sex. The gender differences by various socio-economic factors are also discussed. The socio-economic factors considered include age, education, marital status, children status, work status, employment status, personal income and household type.

In 1999, the distribution of population between males and females was 50:50. In 2004, the ratio had changed to 49:51. This is a reliable outcome, compared to national statistics which show a 50:50 composition of the population between males and females.

For the age analysis, we disaggregated the data into three age groups. The first was 10–14, the second 15–64 and the final was 65 and over. In both 1999 and 2004, the second age group comprised more than 80 per cent of the sample. The proportion of females aged 65 and over increased by two percentage points between 1999 and 2004, from 10 to 12 per cent, while the male proportion remained constant at 8 per cent.

In both surveys, the majority of the sample, 90 per cent, lived in urban areas in 1999 and 92 per cent in 2004. The 1995 and 2000 population and housing census from which the TUS sample is drawn, shows 12 per cent of the population living in rural settlement in 1995 and 10 per cent in 2000.

The survey used seven categories for educational achievement. They are: no education, primary school, middle school, high school, two years of college, four years of university and graduate school. To simplify matters, the descriptive analysis here groups the respondents into three categories. For low education, we include those with no education and those with primary school education; for middle level of education, we include those with middle and high school education; and we include those with college education and above under high level of education. Around 50 per cent of the sample had middle level of education. Between 1999 and 2004, the percentage with college and above education increased for both men and women—from 28 to 36 per cent for men, and from 18 to 26 per cent for women. In both years more men than women—had high education.

Around 60 per cent of the individuals are married. Divorced and widowed men constituted 3 per cent of all men in 1999 and 2004. For women the equivalent figures were 14 per cent in both 1999 and 2004. This is similar to the national statistics, but for a slightly different age group. According to the NSO (NSO, 2000; 2005), in 2000, among those aged 15 and over, married men accounted for 61 per cent, single men 35 per cent and divorced/widowed men 4 per cent. In 2005, the corresponding figures were 35 per cent, 60 per cent, and 5 per cent. Among women, in 2000, 25 per cent were single, 60 per cent were married, and 15 per cent were divorced/widowed. In 2005, the equivalent figures were 25 per cent, 58 per cent, and 16 per cent.

We distinguish between those who have preschool children who are 8 years old or younger, referred to as the "with children" group, and those who do not. Around 20 per cent of men and women reported that they had children in this age group in 1999, while the figures decreased to 15 per cent for men and 14 per cent for women in 2004. This may in part reflect the fall in the fertility rate, which dropped from 1.42 to 1.16 between 1999 and 2004.

The TUS asks respondents if they have worked for pay during the preceding week. The TUS considers those answering "yes" as employed. Among men, 65 per cent responded that they were employed in 1999. In contrast, only 45 per cent of women reported that they were employed. The percentages were slightly higher in 2004, at 67 and 47 per cent respectively.

In 1999, 62 per cent of employed men reported being salary workers and the proportion increased by three percentage points in 2004. In contrast, 58 per cent of female workers reported being salaried in 1999, and the figure increased by 8 percentage points in 2004. As a result, the proportion of women who were salary workers became very similar to that of men. According to the NSO, in 2000 salary workers were 60 per cent of the total female work force, while for males, the equivalent figure was 64 per cent. It increased to 65 per cent for men and 64 per cent for women in 2005.

Unfortunately, we cannot provide analysis by income group for 1999 as data on income are not available for this year. The 2004 TUS collects personal income data in terms of 10 income groups. The first group earns less than $500 per month, the second between $500 and $999, the third $1,000–1,499, the fourth $1,500–1,999, the fifth $2,000–2,499, sixth $2,500–2,999, seventh $3,000–3,499, eighth $3,500–3,999, ninth $4,000–4999 and tenth $5,000 and over. We provide the income distribution of the sample, re-grouping these into five groups. Thirty-four per cent of men and 61 per cent of women had no personal income. Twelve per cent of men and 23 per cent of women had an income less than $1,000 per month; 3 per cent of men and 0.3 per cent of women had an income more than $ 4,000 per month. 99 per cent of women and 91 per cent of men had either no income or an income that was less than $2,999 per month.

For analysis of household composition, three age groups of household members are defined namely: children (Ch; 10–19 years), adult (Ad; 20–59 years) and older adults (Old; 60 years and older). From this, we formulate six household types. They are "Ch+Ad", "Ch+Ad+Old", "Ad", "Ad+Old", "Old" and "Ch+Old". The number of "Ch" is too small to report.

Household types classified as "Ch & Ad" and "Ad" together account for more than 70 per cent of all household types in both 1999 and 2004. The proportion of three-generation households (i.e. "Ch+Ad+Old") decreased between 1999 and 2004, while the proportion of older households increased. The proportion of females in Old households is larger than that of males, and the proportion living in Old households increased between 1999 and 2004 more for women than for men.

Finally, we use the care dependency ratio described in Chapter 1 to give an indication of the need for care. The population and housing censuses of 2000 and 2005 produced by the NSO were used for the calculation of the care dependency ratio. We find that the care dependency ratio is 0.15 in 2000 and 0.18 in 2005. In 2005, the number of children under 12 years old increased by 27 per cent and those aged 65 and over increased by 37 per cent, whereas the number of caregivers increasedby 18 per cent. It is these changes which translate into an increase in the care dependency ratio in 2005.

DEFINING PAID AND UNPAID WORK

For the analysis that follows, paid work includes all the time use activities that are classified under employment including travel for work purposes. In the case of 2004 data, we also included category 611 or "helping for gainful activities". For extended SNA work, the analysis covers household maintenance, person care and the voluntary category as unpaid care work. Person care includes all the activities within family care as well as travel for family care; it also includes community services and help to other households. Household maintenance includes all the activities classified under household care.

Before looking at the time spent on paid and unpaid care work, we present the proportions of time spent on different activities, based on the categories produced by NSO. Figures are percentages of time spent, calculated for a 24-hour period. All activities thus sum to 1,440 minutes.

Between 1999 and 2004, time spent by individuals on personal care and leisure increased. In contrast, time spent on employment and study decreased. There are significant gender differences in the time that is allocated to employment, household care and family care. Men spent 19 per cent and 18 per cent of their time on employment in 1999 and 2004 respectively, while women spent 12 per cent and 11 per cent respectively. For the same years men spent 1 per cent and 2 per cent of their time on household care, while women spent 11 and 10 per cent. Men spent 1 per cent on family care while women spent 3 per cent on family care.

IDENTIFICATION OF KEY DETERMINANTS OF TIME SPENT ON CARE

Tables 5.1 through 5.4 present outcomes of Tobit estimations to identify key independent variables for time spent on unpaid care work and person care. The estimation for unpaid care work and person care is run for both 1999 and 2004 considering variables such as sex, age, age-squared, education, marital status, preschool children in the home, and employment for

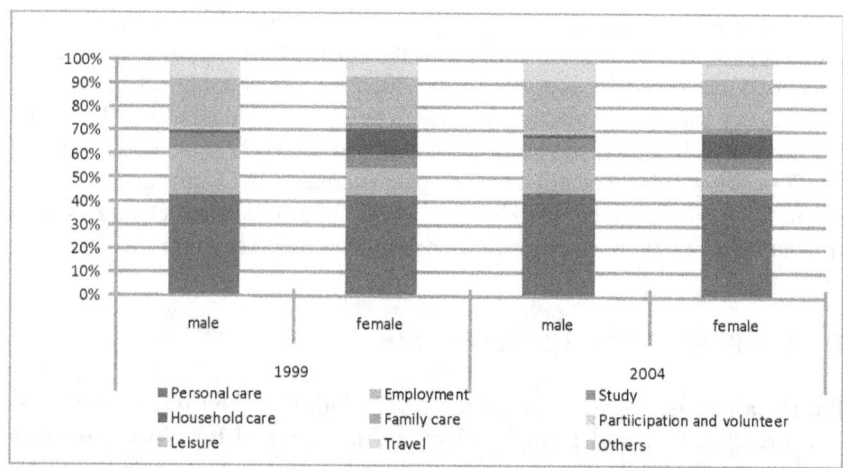

Figure 5.1 Time spent on activities by sex in 1999 and 2004.

both years. "LowEd" is defined as primary school or no education, while "HighEd" is defined as college education or above.

All variables except education are significant factors for time spent on unpaid care work in 1999. Of the discrete variables, being male has the strongest effect, followed by being employed. It appears that being married, having preschool children, and being young increase the time that is spent on unpaid care work while other factors decrease it. All the variables

Table 5.1 Regression Outputs on Duration of Time Spent on Unpaid Care Work, 1999

	Coef.	Std. Err.	t	P>t	95% Conf. Interval	
Male	-228.7	1.2	-181.4	0.000	-231.4	-226.2
Married	85.7	1.7	49.4	0.000	82.3	89.1
Employed	-126.9	1.3	-93.3	0.000	-129.5	-124.2
Childed	93.4	1.5	61.6	0.000	90.4	96.4
LowEd	0.7	1.9	4.1	0.684	-3.0	4.6
HighEd	1.6	1.7	9.3	0.351	-1.8	0.5
Age	15.5	0.2	796.0	0.000	16.1	16.9
Age squared	-0.1	.0	-724.4	0.000	-0.1	-0.1
Constant	-146.4	3.4	-422.3	0.000	153.2	-139.6

Table 5.2 Regression Outputs on Duration of Time Spent on Person Care, 1999

	Coef.	Std. Err.	t	P>t	95% Conf. Interval	
Male	-106.9	1.6	-64.7	0.000	-110.1	-103.6
Married	98.0	2.3	41.7	0.000	93.4	102.6
Employed	-82.5	1.6	-49.5	0.000	-85.7	-79.2
Childed	165.2	1.7	95.3	0.000	161.8	168.6
LowEd	-17.9	2.4	-7.3	0.000	-22.7	-13.1
HighEd	10.2	2.0	4.9	0.000	6.1	14.3
Age	8.8	0.2	30.6	0.000	8.2	9.3
Age squared	-0.09	.0	-30.4	0.000	-0.1	-0.0
Constant	-278.7	5.0	-55.2	0.000	-288.6	-268.8

together explain 48.3 per cent of the variance in the time spent on unpaid care work.

All variables are also found to be statistically significant for time spent on person care. Of the discrete variables, having preschool children has the strongest effect, followed by being male. Being male, being employed, and having minimal education tend to decrease time spent on person care while

Table 5.3 Regression Outputs on Duration of Time Spent on Unpaid Care Work, 2004

	Coef.	Std. Err.	t	P>t	95% Conf. Interval	
Male	-203.2	1.3	-146.6	0.000	-205.9	-200.5
Married	63.6	1.9	33.1	0.000	59.9	67.4
Employed	-127.3	1.5	-83.3	0.000	-130.3	-124.3
Childed	130.3	2.0	63.8	0.000	126.3	134.3
LowEd	1.7	2.2	0.7	0.444	-2.6	6.0
HighEd	3.8	1.7	2.2	0.026	0.4	7.2
Age	16.4	0.2	74.0	0.000	16.0	16.8
Age squared	-1.5	0.0	-64.8	0.000	-1.6	-0.1
Constant	-157.1	3.8	-41.2	0.000	-164.5	-149.6

Table 5.4 Regression Outputs on Duration of Time Spent on Person Care, 2004

	Coef.	Std. Err.	t	P>t	95% Conf. Interval	
Male	-88.2	1.8	-48.3	0.000	-91.8	-84.7
Married	79.7	2.6	29.8	0.000	74.4	84.9
Employed	-90.2	1.9	-46.8	0.000	-93.7	-86.2
Childed	180.7	2.3	77.1	0.000	176.2	185.0
LowEd	-9.8	2.9	-3.3	0.001	-15.5	-4.0
HighEd	9.7	2.1	4.6	0.000	5.6	13.9
Age	8.9	0.3	28.8	0.000	8.3	9.5
Age squared	-0.1	.0	-28.8	0.000	-0.1	-.09
Constant	-256.5	5.5	-46.4	0.000	-267.3	-245.6

other factors increase it. All the variables together explain 21.7 per cent of the variance in the time spent on person care.

In 2004, apart from education, all factors tested for an influence on the allocation of time for unpaid care work are statistically significant. Of the discrete factors, being male remains the strongest factor, followed by having preschool children. Being married, having children, and age tend to increase time spent on unpaid care work while other factors decrease it. All the variables together explain 47.8 per cent of the variance in the time spent on unpaid care work.

All the factors, this time including education, are also found to be significant for influencing the allocation of time on person care in 2004. Of the discrete factors, as in 1999, having preschool children has the strongest influence, followed by being male. Being married, having preschool children, being highly educated, and age tend to increase time spent on person care while other factors decrease it. All the variables together explain 23.1 per cent of the variance in the time spent on person care.

TIME SPENT ON PAID WORK AND UNPAID CARE WORK

This section examines how individuals and households spent time on SNA work and extended SNA work (which includes household maintenance and person care) in 1999 and 2004. The following tables provide percentages of the day reflecting mean population time (MPT) and participation rates (PR).

There are significant gender differences in time spent on paid and unpaid care work. In 1999, men spent 22 per cent of their day on paid work while women spent 13 per cent. Men spent 2 per cent of their day on unpaid care work, while women spent 14 per cent. This means women spent seven

Table 5.5 Time onPaid and Unpaid Care Work by Sex (%), 1999 and 2004

		1999		2004	
		MPT	PR	MPT	PR
Male	SNA work	22	60	21	60
	Household maintenance	1	36	2	37
	Person care	1	15	1	17
Female	SNA work	13	42	12	42
	Household maintenance	11	83	11	82
	Person care	3	40	3	39

times more time on unpaid care work than men did, while the time women spent on paid work was just over 59 per cent of that spent by men. In 2004, both men and women spent slightly reduced time on paid work, although significant gender differences remained. Males spent 3 per cent of a day on unpaid care work while women spent 14 per cent. In addition, men spent 21 per cent of a day on paid work while women spent 12 per cent.

A gendered pattern also exists in the participation rate for paid and unpaid care work. In 2004, more men (60 per cent) than women (42 per cent) participated in paid work while a considerable number of women but fewer men participated in unpaid care work. 82 per cent of women spent some time on household maintenance while only 37 per cent of men did so. In addition, 39 per cent of women and 17 per cent of men spent some time on person care.

Table 5.6 shows time spent on paid and unpaid work in 1999 and 2004 by gender and age group. Several important features emerge from this table. First, there was a significant increase in time spent by young people on household maintenance and person care between 1999 and 2004. In 1999, the time spent and participation rates were small, while in 2004, 23 per cent of males aged between 10 and 14 spent some time on household maintenance, averaging 5 per cent of the day over the male population of this age, while 8 per cent of them spent time on person care, with a mean population time of 3 per cent of the day. In the case of their female counterparts, in 2004, 35 per cent of females aged between 10 and 14 spent time on household maintenance, averaging 10 per cent of the day over the male population of this age, while 10 per cent of them spent time on person care, with a mean population time of 3 per cent of the day. The increases in both the amount of time and the participation rates are due to an increase in their involvement in the activities during the weekends.

Second, apart from the youngest age group, significant gender differences are evident in time spent on paid and unpaid work. Men aged 15 to 64 spent 26 per cent of the day in 1999 and 25 per cent in 2004 on paid work. In contrast, women in the same age group spent 15 per cent in 1999 and 14 per cent in 2004 on paid work. Thus, women in this age group spent 9 percentage points less time than men on paid work in 1999 and 11 percentage points less in 2004. Men in this category spent 2 per cent of their time in both years on unpaid care work, while women spent 15 per cent of their time in both 1999 and 2004. Furthermore, older men spent 12 per cent of their time on paid work and 4 per cent on unpaid care work in 1999 and 2004. In contrast, older women spent 8 per cent of their time on paid work and 13 per cent on unpaid care work in 1999, and 7 and 13 per cent, respectively, in 2004.

Participation rates also reflect gendered patterns for both paid and unpaid care work. Among men, 68 per cent aged 15 to 64 participated in paid work in 2004. The corresponding figure for women is 47 per cent. In terms of participation in household maintenance, although 85 per cent of women aged 15 to 64 participated in 2004, only 37 per cent of men did so. Older women's participation in household maintenance appears to be much higher than that of older men's: 93 per cent of women participated in household maintenance, while only 59 per cent of older men did in 2004.

Table 5.7 shows time spent on paid and unpaid work by gender and education. In 1999, men with a lower education level spent 22 per cent of the day on paid work while women in the same category spent 15 per cent; on unpaid work, the amount of time was 3 and 15 per cent of the day, respectively. Women with a mid-level education spent nine times more time on

Table 5.6 Time on Paid and Unpaid Care Work by Sex and Age Group (%), 1999 and 2004

			1999		2004	
			MPT	PR	MPT	PR
Male	10–14	SNA work	0.1	0	0.1	0.1
		Household maintenance	0.5	1	5	23
		Person care	0.1	0.4	2	8
	15–64	SNA work	26	68	25	68
		Household maintenance	1	36	1	37
		Person care	1	16	1	19
	65+	SNA work	12	49	12	49
		Household maintenance	3	54	3	59
		Person care	1	14	1	15
Female	10–14	SNA work	0.1	0.1	0	0
		Household maintenance	1	3	10	35
		Person care	0.3	0.8	3	10
	15–64	SNA work	15	46	14	47
		Household maintenance	12	87	11	85
		Person care	3	45	4	44
	65+	SNA work	8	37	7	36
		Household maintenance	12	90	12	93
		Person care	1	21	1	21

Table 5.7 Time on Paid and Unpaid Care Work by Sex and Education (%), 1999 and 2004

			1999		2004	
			MPT	PR	MPT	PR
Male	Low	SNA work	22	68	19	67
		Household maintenance	2	54	2	54
		Person care	1	14	1	14
	Middle	SNA work	30	79	28	76
		Household maintenance	1	37	1	41
		Person care	1	18	1	20
	High	SNA work	1	36	1	38
		Household maintenance	3	54	3	59
		Person care	1	21	1	23
Female	Low	SNA work	15	53	12	48
		Household maintenance	13	95	13	95
		Person care	2	25	1	25
	Middle	SNA work	15	49	15	49
		Household maintenance	15	94	14	95
		Person care	4	58	4	54
	High	SNA work	17	51	16	50
		Household maintenance	11	85	10	84
		Person care	5	52	5	51

unpaid work than men with a similar education level, while women with higher education spent over eight times more time on unpaid work than the corresponding men. The gender differences remained similar in 2004. For example, women with a mid-level education spent nine times more time on unpaid care work than men with similar education.

Furthermore, for men, the more educated they were, the more likely they were to participate in paid work. In 1999, 68 per cent of men with a low level of education, 79 per cent for those with a mid-level education, and 77 per cent with higher-level education spent some time on paid work.

Interestingly, even though the amount of time spent by men on person care is the same for all education levels, men with higher education were more likely to be involved in person care than men with lower educational qualifications. Fourteen per cent of men with a low-level education did person care compared to 18 and 21 per cent for those with middle and higher educational qualifications, respectively.

However, men with a low-level education were more involved in household maintenance than men with higher education levels; in 1999, 54 per cent (low), 37 per cent (middle), and 36 per cent (high) spent some time on household maintenance. These patterns remained in 2004.

Women with a mid-level education spent more time on unpaid care work than those with other education levels. In 1999, women with a mid-level education spent 19 per cent of their day on this work, while women with a low level spent 17 per cent, and women with higher education spent 16 per cent on unpaid care work. This difference remained in 2004. Furthermore, it appears that women with higher education spent more time on person care than those with lower education levels. In 1999, minimally educated women spent 2 per cent while mid-level spent 4 per cent and highly educated women spent 5 per cent; in 2004, the corresponding figures are 1, 4 and 5 per cent, respectively. Highly educated women tended to spend less time on household maintenance than those with less educational qualifications. This may be in part because highly educated women can afford to hire helpers for household maintenance or purchase equipment that eases the burden of household maintenance.

Table 5.8 shows time spent on paid and unpaid care work by gender and marital status. In 2004, married men spent more time on paid work than single or divorced/widowed men. Divorced/widowed men appear to have spent more time on unpaid care work than married men. In 2004, married men spent 28 per cent of their time on paid work and 3 per cent on unpaid care work. In contrast, divorced/widowed men spent 17 per cent on paid work and 5 per cent on unpaid care work. Meanwhile, divorced/widowed women spent less time both on paid and unpaid care work than married women. In 2004, married women spent 13 per cent on paid work and 20 per cent on unpaid care work, while divorced/widowed women spent 12 per cent on both paid and unpaid care work.

Table 5.9 shows time spent on paid work and care by gender and children status. Having preschool children meant more time spent on paid work for men, but less time for women. In 2004, men with children spent 32 per cent of their day on paid work, while childless men spent 19 per cent. In the same year, women with children spent 9 per cent of their time on paid work while childless women spent 13 per cent on paid work. Having preschool children also significantly impacted time spent on unpaid work. Women with preschool children spent more time on unpaid work—by 12 percentage points in 1999 and 16 percentage points in 2004—than childless women. The amount of time spent on unpaid

Table 5.8 Time on Paid and Unpaid Care Work by Sex and Marital Status (%), 1999 and 2004

			1999		2004	
			MPT	PR	MPT	PR
Male	Single	SNA work	11	30	11	32
		Household maintenance	1	31	1	30
		Person care	0.5	5	1	6
	Married	SNA work	29	79	28	78
		Household maintenance	1	38	2	41
		Person care	1	21	1	24
	Divorced/ Widowed	SNA work	19	56	17	56
		Household maintenance	4	63	4	71
		Person care	1	14	1	14
Female	Single	SNA work	10	28	11	31
		Household maintenance	2	53	2	48
		Person care	0.3	8	0.3	7
	Married	SNA work	14	48	13	46
		Household maintenance	16	98	15	98
		Person care	4	60	5	59
	Divorced/ Widowed	SNA work	13	45	12	43
		Household maintenance	11	90	11	93
		Person care	1	25	1	23

care work by women with preschool children is more than eight times greater than the time spent by males.

Table 5.10 shows time spent on paid work and unpaid care work by gender and work status. Again, significant gender differences are evident. For women, not being employed means increased time spent on unpaid care work. In 1999, employed women spent 12 per cent of the day on unpaid care work while women who were not employed spent 16 per cent. In 2004, the corresponding figures are 11 and 16 per cent, respectively. In addition, unlike men, for women employment does not necessarily mean a smaller

Table 5.9 Time on Paid and Unpaid Care Work by Sex and Children Status (%), 1999 and 2004

			1999		2004	
			MPT	PR	MPT	PR
Male	With preschool children	SNA work	31	80	32	85
		Household maintenance	1	32	1	36
		Person care	2	38	2	51
	Without preschool children	SNA work	20	56	19	56
		Household maintenance	1	37	1	38
		Person care	1	9	1	11
Female	With preschool children	SNA work	9	34	9	33
		Household maintenance	14	91	14	98
		Person care	10	83	13	98
	Without preschool children	SNA work	14	44	13	43
		Household maintenance	11	81	10	80
		Person care	1	28	1	29

proportion of time spent on unpaid work. In 1999, employed men spent 2 per cent of the day on unpaid care work, while employed women spent 12 per cent on unpaid work. Similar gender differentials are evident in 2004 as well.

Table 5.11 shows the time spent on paid and unpaid care work by household type. There are significant gender differences in terms of time spent on paid and unpaid care work. In 1999, except for individuals in Ad+Old and Old household, all male groups spent only 1 per cent of their time on extended SNA work. Meanwhile, women in all household types spent between 9 and 14 per cent of their time on household care and between 1 and 5 per cent on person care. The gender differences remained significant in 2004.

DISTRIBUTION OF TIME

The distribution of time presented subsequently covers the population aged 15 to 64. It shows the percentage of the male and female population that spent shorter and longer periods of time on unpaid care. For this

Table 5.10 Time on Paid and Unpaid Care Work by Sex and Work Status (%), 1999 and 2004

			1999		2004	
			MPT	PR	MPT	PR
Male	Working	SNA work	34	89	32	86
		Household maintenance	1	36	1	38
		Person care	1	17	1	20
	Not working	SNA work	1	7	1	8
		Household maintenance	2	38	2	38
		Person care	1	11	1	12
Female	Working	SNA work	28	86	26	83
		Household maintenance	10	89	9	87
		Person care	2	37	2	36
	Not working	SNA work	1	5	1	6
		Household maintenance	12	62	12	79
		Person care	4	42	4	42

distribution it would be ideal to use full minutes; however, this analysis uses a 24-hour approach for two reasons. The first reason is the non-availability of data on simultaneous activities for 1999, despite the fact that the NSO collected data on both main and simultaneous activities in that year. Second, there are very small differences between time spent on main and all activities for 2004. For example, in 2004, the time differences are 0.09 minutes for production activities, 0.45 for household maintenance, and 0.01 for personal care for males. For females, the average time difference between main activities and main and simultaneous activities combined are 0.75, 1.17, and 0.01 minutes, respectively. For comparative purpose, this analysis therefore focuses on the main activities, with the total amount of time spent on these activities equalling 24 hours.

Figure 5.2 shows the distribution of time spent on unpaid care work by sex in 1999. According to the data, 54 per cent of males spent almost no time on unpaid care work. At the other end of the scale, 1.5 per cent of females spent more than 12 hours on unpaid care work, while no males did so.

Figure 5.3 shows the distribution of time on person care in 1999. Almost 83 per cent of males and 55 per cent of females spent no time on person

Republic of Korea 133

Table 5.11 Time on Work and Care by Household Type (%), 1999 and 2004

		1999			2004		
		SNA work	Household maintenance	Person care	SNA work	Household maintenance	Person care
Male	Ch+Ad	18 47	1 29	1 10	17 47	1 30	1 13
	Ch+Ad+Old	16 46	1 30	1 12	14 44	1 31	1 15
	Ad	29 76	1 39	1 20	27 73	1 40	1 22
	Ad+Old	23 65	2 42	1 17	22 65	2 42	1 15
	Old	14 55	3 61	1 12	13 54	4 64	1 14
	Ch+Old	5 20	1 40	1 11	4 16	1 37	1 10
Female	Ch+Ad	11 35	9 73	2 36	10 34	9 70	2 40
	Ch+Ad+Old	11 39	9 76	2 30	9 33	9 72	2 35
	Ad	15 46	13 92	5 52	15 48	11 89	5 46
	Ad+Old	14 48	12 88	3 38	13 46	13 88	3 34
	Old	12 49	14 97	2 18	10 46	14 97	1 18
	Ch+Old	6 25	9 80	1 30	5 21	10 80	1 27

care. Meanwhile, 0.7 per cent of males and 2.5 per cent of females spent more than 6 hours per day on person care.

Figure 5.4 shows the distribution of time on unpaid care work in 2004. Over 51 per cent of males but around 13 per cent of females spent no time on unpaid care work. Meanwhile, no males and 1 per cent of females spent more than 12 hours on unpaid care work

In 2004, 80 per cent of males and 56 per cent of females spent no time on person care while 1 per cent of males and 3 per cent of females spent more than 6 hours on person care.

VALUATION AND COMPARISON OF UNPAID CARE WORK

This section discusses the value of unpaid care work, comparing it to various economic measures. This discussion utilises the average earnings and generalist approaches. Ideally, the average earnings approach uses average earnings for all people in the economy. We use earnings of all employed people (i.e. including the self-employed, own account and employers alongside employees) as well as earnings for all employees (i.e. those earning wages or salaries). The all employees approach uses the average earnings for all paid

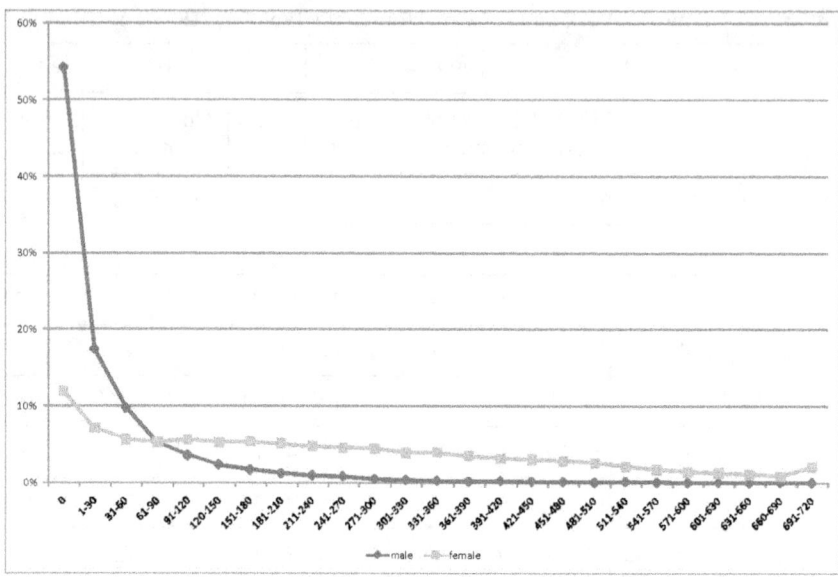

Figure 5.2 Distribution of time spent on unpaid care work by sex, 1999.

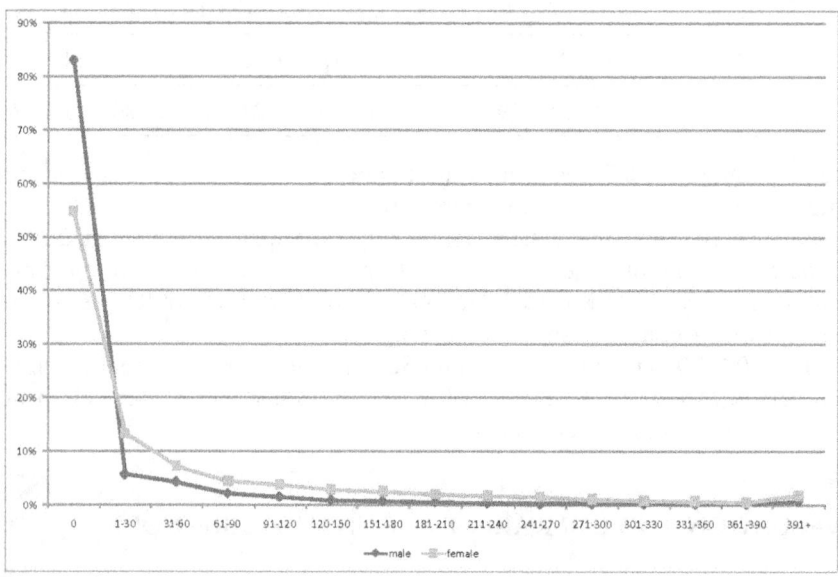

Figure 5.3 Distribution of time spent on person care by sex, 1999.

employees. The all employed approach uses the average earnings for self-employed, own account workers and employees. Three national datasets are designed to collect information on earnings: the Wage Structure Survey

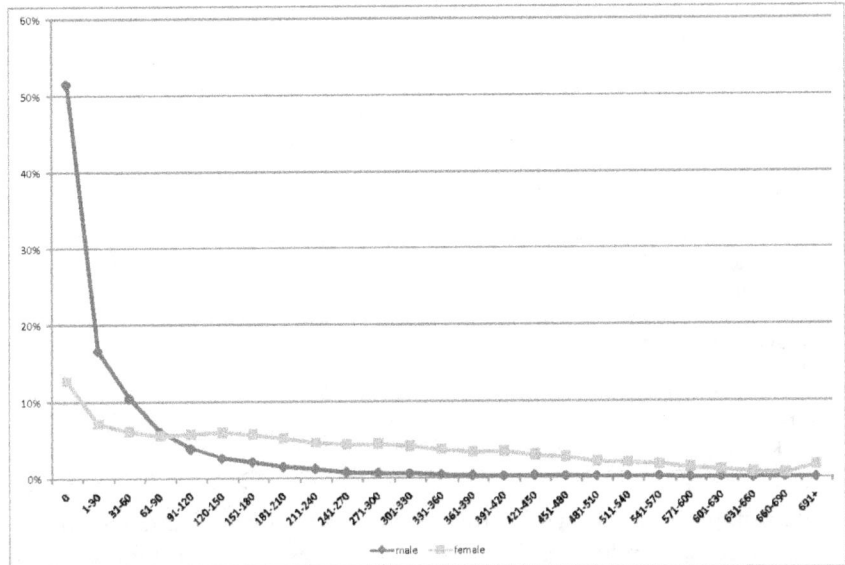

Figure 5.4 Distribution of time spent on person care work by sex, 2004.

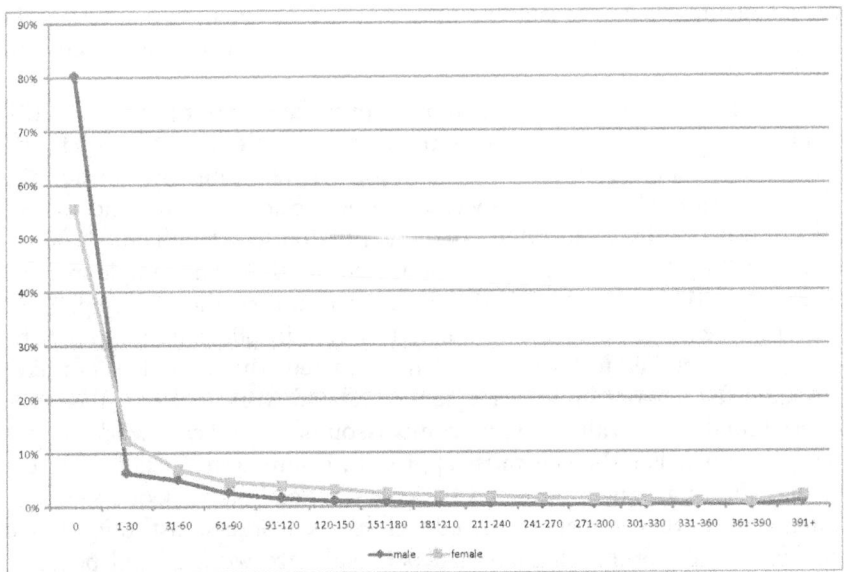

Figure 5.5 Distribution of time spent on person care, 2004.

of the Ministry of Labour, the Economically Active Population Survey of the NSO, and the Korean Labour and Income Panel Survey (KLIP) of the Korean Labour Institute. The first of these collects wage information for

Table 5.12 Unpaid Care Work and Person Care as Percentage of GDP: Different Approaches

	Unpaid care work			Person care		
	Male	Female	Total	Male	Female	Toatl
Average earnings for all employed	6	24	29	2	6	8
Average wages of all employees	5	24	29	2	6	8
Average generalist wage	-	-	18	-	-	5
Average domestic worker wage	-	-	19	-	-	5

regular employees who work in workplaces with five or more employees, excludes certain industries including the domestic service industry, and does not collect earnings information by occupation in detail; these are all disadvantages in light of the current discussion. The second survey does not collect earnings data for self-employed or wage information by occupation in detail, which are also disadvantages given the purpose of the current analysis.

Thus the KLIP seems to be the most appropriate for our purposes. KLIP is a longitudinal study of representative samples of Korean households and individuals living in urban areas. It is constructed annually to track the characteristics of households as well as economic activities, income, expenditure, job training, education, and social activities of individuals. Initiated in 1998, the ninth wave was conducted in 2006. The sample in 1998 included 5,000 households. KLIP collects wage information for employees, self-employed, and personal accounts. Moreover, it collects earnings data by occupation detailed to three digits. Unfortunately, the KLIP does not have any data for females in domestic service-related work in 1999. Thus, the current analysis on valuation and comparison of unpaid care work focuses on 2004 only. For the generalist approach, occupations included for the calculation of average wages and the codes are as follows: Code 411: personal services related workers includes childcare workers, institution-based personal care workers, home-based personal care workers and personal care and related workers; Code 421: cooks including head cooks, restaurant cooks, fast-food restaurant cooks and tea cooks; Code 911: domestic and related helpers, cleaners and launderers, include char workers, building cleaners, cleaners in hotels and restaurants, vehicle and related cleaners and hand launderers and pressers.

For the domestic wage approach, wages of domestic and related helpers, cleaners and launderers are considered.

Table 5.13 Total Value of Unpaid Care Work and Person by Year (Thousand Million Won): Different Approaches

	Unpaid care work			Person care		
	Male	Female	Total	Male	Female	Toatl
Average earnings for all employed	46,530	183,659	225,125	18,684	43,240	59,335
Average wages of all employees	41,297	185,944	222,685	16,583	43,777	58,692
Average generalist wage	-	-	138,086	-	-	36,395
Average domestic worker wage	-	-	144,861	-	-	38,180

Table 5.12 shows the value of unpaid care work and personal care as a percentage of gross domestic product (GDP), which was 779,380,000 million won in 2004.

The value of unpaid care work done by males was equivalent to 6 per cent of GDP using the all employed approach. The value of person care by males was 2 per cent. In contrast, the value of unpaid care work by females was 24 per cent and for person care it was 6 per cent. In total, the value of unpaid care work ranged from 18 per cent of GDP using the generalist approach, to 29 per cent using all employed approach in 2004. The value of work on personal care ranged from 5 to 7 per cent depending on the approach used.

Table 5.13 shows the value of unpaid care work and person care in absolute terms. The value of unpaid care work is estimated at between 41,297,404 million won and 225,124,975 million. The value of person care is between 16,582,741 million won and 59,335,264 million won.

We can also compare the value of unpaid care work with tax revenues. Taxes in Korea comprise national and local taxes. National taxes are divided into internal taxes, customs duties, and three earmarked taxes; the local taxes include province taxes and city and county taxes. The internal taxes consist of direct and indirect taxes. Direct taxes include income tax, corporation tax, inheritance and gift tax, and comprehensive real estate holding tax. Indirect tax includes value-added tax, special excise tax, liquor tax, stamp tax, securities transaction tax and transportation tax. Of these ten taxes, the income tax, corporation tax, and value added tax make up the bulk of the Korean tax revenue. We use both direct and total tax for comparison. In 2004, direct tax was 49,806,900 million won and total gross tax was 151,997,400 million won (NSO 2007).

The value of unpaid care work is clearly larger than that of direct tax regardless of the approach used. Even the value of personal care exceeds the value of direct tax for two approaches. The value of unpaid care work exceeds that of total taxes in both the all employed and all employees approaches.

To compare the value of unpaid care work with the value of paid work, we calculate the total wages earned by paid employees. In other words, we exclude self-employed and unpaid family workers. For the volume of earnings of paid employees, we multiply the total earnings calculated from NSO data by the number of the paid employees. In 2004, earnings for all paid work equaled 131,300,600 million won for males and 37,078,900 million won for females, for a total of 168,379,600 million won.

The value of unpaid care work done by males was 28 per cent of total earnings when using the all employed approach. The value of person care work done by males was 11 per cent of all paid work using both the all employed and all employees approaches and 10 per cent using the all employed approach. The value of person care by females was 26 per cent of all paid work in economy using both the all employed and all employees approaches. The value of unpaid care work done by women is greater than the total value of paid work done in the economy by around 10 percentage points.

Social services such as education, health and social welfare are managed and delivered by national and provincial sphere of governments. Unfortunately, however, a source on provincial government's expenditure on the care-related personnel expenditure is not available. Thus, our comparison has to focus on care-related personnel expenditure of central government which underestimates the total value of government expenditure on care-related personnel expenditure. For education, we aggregate the personnel expenditures of national and public schools, Ministry of Education and educational support institutions under the Ministry (17,780,731 million won) and the personnel expenditure of Ministry of Health and Social Welfare (172,189 million won) to arrive at a total of 17,952,920 million won.

We find that the value of unpaid care work could be more than twelve times that of national government's social services. Even with the generalist wage approach, it is more than seven times the value of government social services. The value of person care could also be more than three times that of government social services, using the average earnings for all employed approach.

We can also compare the value of unpaid care work with remuneration of paid workers in care-related occupations as recoded in the Economically Active Population Survey of the NSO. We include all occupations classified under the personal services related workers (occupation code 411) and domestic and related helpers, clearners and launders (occupation code 911). For the volume of earnings of paid care workers, we multiply the total earnings by the number of the paid care workers, as reported by the NSO. In 2004, total paid care workers' earnings equalled 5,108,098 million won. For women it was 1,565,329 million won while for men it was 3,542,770 million won.

Table 5.14 Comparison of Total Annual Hours Spent on Paid Work, Unpaid Care Work and Person Care

	Male	Female	Total
Paid work	39,359,838,761	23,070,524,905	62,213,471,662
Unpaid care work	5,328,697,339	26,563,416,520	32,105,672,478
Person care	2,139,708,584	6,253,906,724	8,461,960,188

We find that the value of unpaid care work could be more than 43 times that of paid care workers. Even with the generalist wage, it is more than 27 times the value of paid care workers. In particular, the value of unpaid care work by women could be more than 117 times that of female paid care workers. The value of person care by women could also be more than 27 times that of paid care workers, using the average earnings for all employed and employees approach.

Finally, Table 5.14 shows total hours spent on unpaid care work, person care, and paid work for both males and females. In 2004, the number of hours females spent on paid work equalled 59 per cent of those males spent. The number of hours males spent on unpaid care work equalled only 20 per cent of those females spent. Males spent 34 per cent of the number of hours spent by females on personal care. Overall, the total hours spent on unpaid care work equalled 51 per cent of total hours spent on paid work.

KEY FINDINGS

The analysis of the TUS data relating to time spent on paid and unpaid care work in 1999 and 2004 highlights several features.

- There are significant gender differences in time spent on paid work and care, in that men are more likely to participate in paid work and to spend more time on it, while the opposite pattern holds in respect of unpaid care work. Overall, women spent time more than four times more time on unpaid care work than men while they spent around approximately 57 per cent of the time spent by men on paid work.
- Apart from the youngest age group, 10–14 years, there are significant gender differences in time spent on paid and unpaid work. Among those aged between 15 and 64 years, while men spent considerably larger amounts of time on paid work, women spent similar amounts of time on paid and unpaid care work. The older men are likely to spend time on paid work while the counterpart women did so for unpaid care work.
- There are also significant gender differences in time spent on paid and unpaid care work by education. For example, in 1999 women

with low educational qualification spent about five times more time on unpaid care work than men with a similar level of education; women with a middle level of education spent nine times more time on unpaid work than men with similar education; and those with high education spent eight times more on unpaid care work than their male counterparts. These features remained similar in 2004. In addition, for men, the more educated they are, the more likely they were to participate in paid work, and men with low education were more involved in household maintenance than men with higher education. Furthermore, women with middle education spent the largest amount of time on unpaid care work. Women with high education spent more time on person care than those with lower education levels. Finally, highly educated women tend to spent less time on household maintenance than those with lower education.

- Married individuals spent more on paid work than single, divorced or widowed individuals. Divorced or widowed men appear to spend more time on unpaid care work than married men. Married women spent the longest time on unpaid care work. Divorced/widowed women spent less time both on paid and unpaid care work than married women.
- Having preschool children meant more time spent on paid work for men, but less time spent on paid work for women. Furthermore, women with preschool children spent more time than childless women on unpaid care work by 12 per cent in 1999 and 16 per cent in 2004.
- Employed women spent less time on unpaid care work than women who were not employed. Nevertheless, employed women spent considerably more time on unpaid care work than their male counterparts.
- Among those aged between 15 and 64 years, men spent on average 25 per cent of their day on paid work, 3 per cent on unpaid care work and 72 per cent on non-productive activities during a day. In contrast, women spent 15 per cent on unpaid care work, 16 per cent on paid work and 69 per cent on non-productive activities. Between 1999 and 2004, both men and women spent increased time on non-productive activities. Men spent increased time on unpaid care work and decreased time on paid work, while women spent decreased time on both unpaid care and paid work.
- The value of unpaid care work is equivalent to 29 per cent of GDP using the all employed approach and 18 per cent using the domestic worker approach. The value of person care is 8 per cent using the all employed approach and 5 per cent using the domestic worker approach. Furthermore, we found that the value of unpaid care work is larger than that of direct tax regardless of the approach used. The value of unpaid care work exceeds that of total tax using both the "all employed" and "all employees" approaches. In addition, the value of

person care is 35 per cent of the total value of the paid economy when using both all employed approaches and 22 per cent, using generalist approach. The value of unpaid care work far exceeds the value of central government expenditure on care-related personnel and the remuneration of paid care workers. Finally, we found that the total hours spent on unpaid care work are 51 per cent of total hours spent on paid work.

REFERENCES

National Statistics Office. 2000. *Social Statistics Survey*. http://www.kosis.kr/index.html, accessed on 20 July 2007.
National Statistics Office. 2005. *Social Statistics Survey*. http://www.kosis.kr/index.html, accessed on 20 July 2007.
National Statistics Office. 2007. *Social Statistics Survey*. http://www.kosis.kr/index.html, accessed on 20 July 2007.

6 Analysis of Time Use Surveys on Work and Care in Japan

Yuko Tamiya and Masato Shikata

INTRODUCTION

This chapter analyses time use surveys carried out in Japan, focussing on how people distribute their time between work and care. The Ministry of Internal Affairs and Communications has carried out the Survey on Time Use and Leisure Activities (*Shakai Seikatsu Kihon Chōsa*) every five years from 1976. Using this time survey, we firstly analyse how people spend their time on paid and unpaid work by sex, age, household type, work status and household income. Secondly, we examine how the amount of time Japanese women and men spent in child and elderly care changed between 1991 and 2006. Furthermore, we discuss how these changes may have been influenced by childcare and elderly care policy in this period.

The Survey on Time Use and Leisure Activities (STULA) aims to obtain comprehensive data on daily patterns of time allocation. The latest survey (the seventh) was conducted in 2006. From the 2001 survey (the sixth), Questionnaire B (which uses the post-coding approach) was introduced in order to obtain more detailed results concerning people's time allocation. The pre-coded form used in former surveys was retained and named Questionnaire A. Therefore, from 2001 respondents were divided into two groups. The first group, which comprised the majority of the total sample, answered Questionnaire A while the second much smaller group answered Questionnaire B.

The sample consists of around 70,000 to 100,000 households, covering approximately 200,000 to 250,000 total household members. All persons aged ten and over (15 and over up to the 1991 survey) in the sample households are asked to respond to the survey. The respondents are asked to report their time use on two consecutive days during nine days in September or October.

In Questionnaire A, the kinds of activities are classified into twenty categories. In Questionnaire B, the respondents record their activities by 15-minute intervals, and the activities are subsequently classified into sixty-two categories during tabulation. In this chapter, we collapse these sixty-two categories into ten categories in order to compare the results with those of other countries covered in this book.

In the first half of our analysis, we utilise the data of Questionnaire B in the micro data set from the 2001 STULA.[1] The second half of our analysis uses data from Questionnaire A from the surveys carried out from 1991 to 2006. The data were weighted by region, sex and age.

GENDER DISTRIBUTION OF PAID AND UNPAID WORK IN JAPAN: ANALYSIS OF THE MICRO DATA IN THE 2001 TIME USE SURVEY

Distribution of Time Spent on Paid and Unpaid Work by Respondent Attributes

In the analysis in this section, the daily mean population time is presented for each of the ten categories of activity presented in Chapter 1. We also present an analysis which classifies the activities into broader categories of paid and unpaid work. We define paid work according to the narrow production boundary of the System of National Accounts (SNA). We define unpaid care (UCW) as activities in the categories of household maintenance, care of persons and community services.

Table 6.1 shows the daily mean population time spent by males and females on each of the ten categories of activity. The male–female differential

Table 6.1 Distribution of Activities Over the Day by Sex

	Male		Female	
Activity category	Minutes	%	Minutes	%
Paid work	337	23.4%	166	11.5%
Non-establishment work	1	0.1%	0	0.0%
Household maintenance	45	3.2%	218	15.2%
Care of persons	8	0.6%	26	1.8%
Community service	5	0.4%	4	0.3%
Learning	70	4.9%	67	4.6%
Social & cultural	93	6.5%	89	6.2%
Mass media use	175	12.1%	157	10.9%
Personal care	674	46.8%	682	47.3%
Other	31	2.1%	31	2.2%
Total	1440	100.0%	1440	100.0%

was large in respect of time spent on paid work, household maintenance and care of persons. While males spent 337 minutes on paid work, twice as long as females (166 minutes), they spent less than one hour on household maintenance and care of persons combined. Females spent 218 minutes on household maintenance and 26 minutes on care of persons. Mass media use shows the next biggest contrast in time use between males and females, with males spending 18 minutes longer (175 minutes) than females (157 minutes).

If we group the relevant items in Table 6.1 into UCW and SNA work, we find that females spent 17 per cent of the day on UCW and 12 per cent on SNA work, males spent only 4 per cent on the former and approximately one-fourth of the day on the latter.

Table 6.2 shows time spent on UCW and SNA work by sex and age. Females in every age group spent more than males on UCW, while males spent more time than females on SNA work. Although the male–female differential in SNA work was relatively small among those under 18 years of age, in other age groups males spent approximately twice the amount of time spent by females. As for UCW, the difference in time use was considerable among those between the ages of 18 and 64.

Table 6.3 shows time spent on UCW and SNA work by sex and marital status. Regardless of marital status, females spent more time on UCW and males spent more time on SNA work. This tendency was especially strong among married males and females. Married males spent 65 minutes (5 per cent of the day) on UCW, while married females spent 344 minutes (24 per cent). Married males spent 398 minutes (28 per cent) on SNA work, while married females spent 167 minutes (12 per cent).

Table 6.4 shows time spent on UCW and SNA work by sex and presence of children of different ages. Regardless of the presence and age of children, females spent more time on UCW while males spent more time on SNA work. Those who had children under 7 years of age spent much more time

Table 6.2 Time Spent on Paid and Unpaid Work by Age Group and Sex

	Male				Female			
	10–17	18–49	50–64	65+	10–17	18–49	50–64	65+
UCW	18	54	60	96	34	270	301	244
Of which: Care of persons	0	10	6	11	1	44	13	12
SNA work	13	436	410	147	6	232	204	56
Of which: Paid work	13	436	408	145	6	232	203	55

Table 6.3 Time Spent on Paid and Unpaid Work by Marital Status and Sex

	Male			Female		
	Single	Married	Widowed/ Divorced	Single	Married	Widowed/ Divorced
UCW	39	65	107	79	344	203
Of which: Care of persons	1	12	5	2	42	9
SNA work	243	398	236	188	167	120
Of which: Paid work	243	396	235	188	167	120

Table 6.4 Time Spent on Paid and Unpaid Work by Presence of Children and Sex

	Male			Female		
	No children	7–17 with	<7 with	No children	7–17 with	<7 with
UCW	64	34	79	234	195	405
Of which: Care of persons	5	3	33	9	11	120
SNA work	338	291	423	189	138	121
Of which: Paid work	337	291	422	189	138	120

Table 6.5 Time Spent on Paid and Unpaid Work by Work Status and Sex

	Male		Female	
	Employed	Not employed	Employed	Not employed
UCW	53	74	218	277
Of which: Care of persons	9	7	16	35
SNA work	472	9	334	6
Of which: Paid work	471	8	333	6

than those who had children aged between 7 and 17, not only on care of persons, including childcare, but also on UCW as a whole, and this applied to both males and females. In contrast, while females with children aged 7 to 17 spent more time on SNA work than those with children under 7 years of age, the opposite holds true for males.

Table 6.5 shows time spent on UCW and SNA work by sex and work status. Those who were not employed spent more time on UCW than those employed, and this applied to both males and females. The difference between males and females in the time spent on UCW was about four times in every case, which was much more evident than in the case of SNA work.

Table 6.6 shows time spent on UCW and SNA work by sex and household income. Regardless of annual income, females spent more time on UCW and males spent more time on SNA work. There was a tendency for both males and females to spend less time on UCW and more time on SNA work as their household income increases. However, this tendency was not observed in respect of care of persons.

Regression Analysis

Table 6.7 shows coefficients and standard errors (in parentheses under the coefficients) of a regression analysis conducted unpaid care work. The

Table 6.6 Time Spent on Paid and Unpaid Work by Household Income and Sex

	0–299	300–499	500–699	700–999	1000+
Male					
UCW	72	73	51	50	45
Of which: Care of persons	6	12	9	8	4
SNA work	240	332	364	379	393
Of which: Paid work	239	331	363	379	393
Female					
UCW	242	276	247	235	232
Of which: Care of persons	18	38	26	27	16
SNA work	152	159	152	188	198
Of which: Paid work	152	159	152	188	197

Table 6.7 Regression Results on Duration of Time Spent on Unpaid Care Work

	Male & Female		Male		Female	
Male	−276.2	***				
	(3.93)					
Married	115.1	***	0.1		217.3	***
	(7.02)		(9.67)		(9.21)	
Divorced/widowed	80.4	***	72.1	***	132.5	***
	(10.57)		(16.80)		(12.74)	
With child under 6	112.2	***	92.2	***	136.2	***
	(6.12)		(8.98)		(7.66)	
With old over 65	−8.9	*	−25.3	***	−1.4	
	(4.38)		(6.70)		(5.32)	
Student	−24.5	*	−8.0		−19.5	
	(10.16)		(14.38)		(12.69)	
Low education	−18.4	**	−20.2	*	−18.7	*
	(5.94)		(8.77)		(7.37)	
High education	10.5		26.0	***	12.5	*
	(4.61)		(6.66)		(5.84)	
Low income	12.4	*	18.0	*	3.7	
	(5.35)		(7.90)		(6.59)	
High income	−10.7	+	−24.1	**	1.9	
	(5.52)		(8.08)		(6.86)	
Age	10.3	***	3.4	+	13.2	***
	(1.28)		(1.81)		(1.63)	
Age squared	−0.1	***	0.0		−0.1	***
	(0.01)		(0.02)		(0.02)	
Saturday	50.0	***	69.6	***	36.0	***
	(4.65)		(6.92)		(5.72)	
Sunday	73.5	***	122.6	***	34.9	***
	(4.64)		(6.86)		(5.73)	
Constant	−80.7	**	−181.9	***	−187.6	***
	(25.05)		(35.56)		(31.71)	

***P-value<0.001, **P-value<0.01, *P-value<0.05, + P-value<0.1

subjects of analysis were males and females between the ages of 15 and 64. We set up three models, male, female and male and female combined using a Tobit estimation. As demographic explanatory variables, we used the dummy variables of sex, co-residing with a child aged under 6, and co-residing with an elderly person aged 65 or over, the category variable of marital status, and age and the square of age. For marital status, we observed the effect of married and divorced/widowed, using single as reference category. As socio-economic explanatory variables, we used the category variables of being a student, educational achievement, and household income, and the variable of the day of the week for which the survey was conducted. For academic achievement, we observed the effect of university, junior college and junior high school, using high school as reference category.

The analysis shows that for marital status, the time spent on UCW became significantly longer for those who were married in the case of females, but this effect was not observed for males. Further, living with children younger than 6 years of age significantly lengthened the time spent on UCW of both males and females. In contrast, living with elderly persons aged 65 years and over significantly shortened the time spent on UCW in the case of males, but had no significant effect for females.

As for education and household income, while the time spent on UCW became longer for both males and females as their educational standard rose, it was shortened only for males when household income increased.

Table 6.8 shows the results of an analysis focussing on the time spent on care of persons, conducted using the same method as for UCW.

The male and female combined model shows that the time spent on care of persons was significantly shortened for males. Further, time spent on care of persons was longer for those married and divorced/widowed in comparison with single people. Time spent on care of persons also became longer when living with children. These results were similar to those produced by the separate analyses by gender. For education, household income and days of the week, results of the analyses differed between males and females. Thus while no significant effect was observed for males, time spent on care of persons became significantly longer for females when their educational achievement was high. In contrast, for household income, while no significant effect was observed for females, time spent on care of persons became shorter for males when their income was high. Additionally, while no significant difference for care of persons was observed between weekdays and weekends in the case of females, time spent on care of persons became significantly longer for weekends compared with weekdays in the case of males.

Table 6.9 shows the result of the Tobit estimation of time spent on childcare, conducted using the same method as the preceding analyses. Here the targets of analysis were males and females living with children under 10 years of age. This age cut-off was chosen in order to obtain large enough samples

Table 6.8 Regression Results on Duration of Time Spent on Care of Persons: Males and Females Aged 15–64

	Male & Female		Male		Female	
Male	-102.0	***				
	(5.87)					
Married	193.1	***	140.3	***	223.1	***
	(13.47)		(21.40)		(17.02)	
Divorced/widowed	145.2	***	89.7	**	181.4	***
	(17.91)		(34.24)		(21.29)	
With child under 6	227.5	***	228.0	***	234.9	***
	(7.68)		(13.73)		(9.23)	
With old over 65	-3.6	*	-11.0		3.8	
	(6.36)		(11.67)		(7.45)	
Student	-29.4)	*	-36.4		-17.1	
	(20.27)		(32.61)		(25.74)	
Low education	14.8	+	22.8		9.4	
	(8.43)		(14.34)		(10.12)	
High education	25.9		14.3		34.1	***
	(6.31)		(10.87)		(7.64)	
Low income	-7.3		-7.1		-6.8	
	(8.12)		(14.22)		(9.64)	
High income	-13.3		-26.3	+	-8.4	
	(8.23)		(14.46)		(9.82)	
Age	0.1		-4.8		3.8	
	(2.04)		(3.38)		(2.52)	
Age squared	0.0		0.1		-0.1	*
	(0.02)		(0.04)		(0.03)	
Saturday	23.5	***	74.4	***	-0.1	
	(6.69)		(12.39)		(7.87)	
Sunday	40.8	***	119.5	***	-2.1	
	(6.64)		(12.21)		(7.94)	
Constant	-329.7	***	-370.3	***	-395.0	***
	(41.00)		(68.18)		(51.21)	

***P-value<0.001, **P-value<0.01, *P-value<0.05, + P-value<0.1

for the analysis. Variables used were single parent (dummy variable), the age of the youngest child, education (category variable), household income (category variable), Saturday/Sunday (category variable), number of children under 10 years of age, number of members of household aged ten and over, and employment status (dummy variable). Single parents are defined as those who were unmarried and had children younger than 10 years of age.

Single mothers spent less time on childcare than do married mothers. Time spent on childcare became longer for both males and females when

Table 6.9 Regression Results on Duration of Time Spent on Child Care: Co-residence with Own Child Aged Under 10

	Male		Female	
Single parent	57.7		-53.8	+
	(80.5)		(30.7)	
Age of youngest child	-28.2	***	-26.6	***
	(3.4)		(2.0)	
Low education	24.8		-49.9	*
	(31.4)		(21.6)	
High education	37.5	*	21.5	*
	(15.2)		(9.9)	
Low income	-34.2		-11.1	
	(23.2)		(14.9)	
High income	4.8		-4.4	
	(32.6)		(20.4)	
Saturday	32.3	+	-28.1	*
	(19.2)		(11.8)	
Sunday	46.3	*	-62.5	***
	(20.5)		(12.2)	
Working	-122.5	***	-67.4	***
	(17.0)		(12.1)	
Number of people<10	3.4		-3.6	
	(10.8)		(7.5)	
Number of people>=10	-36.6	**	-12.7	*
	(11.0)		(6.1)	
Constant	143.2	***	264.5	***
	(38.6)		(23.4)	

***P-value<0.001, **P-value<0.01, *P-value<0.05, + P-value<0.1

they were highly educated. Household income did not have a significant effect. As for days of the week, while time spent on childcare became longer on Saturday/Sunday for males, it became shorter for females. With regard to the characteristics of children no significant effect of the number of children younger than 10 years was observed on time spent. Time spent on childcare decreased when the number of household members aged 10 and older increased, which suggests that an increase in the number of household members capable of performing childcare shortened time spent on that activity for individuals. Finally, as expected, time spent on childcare decreased for both males and females when they were working.

Review of the Analysis

From the results of the preceding analysis, we observed the following tendencies in time spent on paid and unpaid work and participation in these activities. Females spent more time on unpaid work and males on paid work, regardless of their age, marital status, presence of children, age of children, employment status, household income or household composition. Time spent on care of persons was significantly shorter for males than females even after controlling for their attributes, which was confirmed by the result of the regression analysis. Further, the participation rate in care of persons was higher for females (females 19.5%, males 8.5%), and the participation rate in paid work was higher for males (females 37.1%, males 58.3%).

Examining the different attributes, we saw that the male–female differential was small among those aged under 18 years of age.

In terms of marital status, the tendency for females to spend more time on UCW and males on SNA work was prominent among those who were married. Significantly more time was spent on care of persons by the married and divorced or widowed, which was confirmed by the result of the regression analysis. As for UCW, the time spent on this became significantly longer for married females, but this effect was not observed among males.

The result of the analysis in terms of the presence of children aged under 18 years and the age of children was that both males and females spent more time on UCW and care of persons, and participated more in care of persons when they have children under 7 years of age (females 72.3%, males 34.4%) than when they had children aged 7 to 17 (females 23.9%, males 4.9%).

Both males and females who were not employed spent more time on UCW than those who were employed. The male–female differential in time spent on UCW was about four times in each case, and larger than the differential in time spent on SNA work. The participation rate in care of persons was higher for females who were not employed (23.3%) than those who were employed (16.6%). This rate was lower for males even when they were not employed (6.2%) and somewhat higher among those who were employed (9.4%).

Although both males and females showed a tendency to spend less time on UCW as their income increased, there was no such tendency observed in childcare and elderly care. The participation rate in care of persons was low among those whose annual income was less than three million yen, for males (6.6%) and females (14.6%) alike, but above that income level the participation rate decreased as annual income increased. In the regression analysis no significant effect was observed among females for household income, but time spent on care of persons and UCW was shortened for males when their income was high.

The regression analysis shows that both males and females spent significantly more time on care of persons when they co-resided with children younger than 6 years old. Further, co-residing with children aged under 6 significantly lengthened the time spent on UCW for both males and females, and co-residing with elderly persons aged 65 or over significantly shortened the time spent on UCW by males, but no significant effect was observed among females. From these results, we can consider that three-generation households reduce the burden of childcare on males through the older people assuming some of the UCW burden, rather than reducing the UCW burden of females.

TRENDS IN THE DAILY PROVISION OF CHILDCARE AND ELDERLY CARE AND THE INFLUENCE OF SOCIAL POLICY IN JAPAN

In this second half of the chapter we examine how the amount of time Japanese men and women spent in childcare and elderly care had changed between 1986 and 2006. Furthermore, we discuss how these changes may have been influenced by childcare and elderly care policy in this period.

In the following analysis, we use the data from Questionnaire A for 1986 to 2006 as these data retain the conventional precoding survey method, allowing comparison of more recent surveys with past ones. As noted before, in Questionnaire A, activities are classified into twenty categories. In the following analysis, we cluster these into five larger categories.

Time Spent on Childcare

In this section, we first draw on comparative data to establish the special characteristics of Japan regarding time spent on childcare for families with at least one child. Next, we examine long-term changes in the amount of time spent in caring for children under 6 years of age by sex of caregiver, household type and mother's employment status.

Table 6.10 shows a twelve-country comparison of daily time use by married couples with at least one child aged 6 or under (given as the weekly average for each of the categories in the original data). The Japanese data

Table 6.10 Twelve-country Comparison of Daily Time Use Among Married Couples with at Least One Child Aged 6 or Under

	Country	Sleep, personal care and meals	Employment and related travel	Housework, shopping and elderly care	Child care	Leisure, study and other
			Mothers			
Married couple with youngest child aged 0–6	Belgium	648	158	206	114	314
	Estonia	623	133	236	159	289
	Finland	627	148	198	154	311
	France	699	146	225	117	253
	Germany	651	81	218	138	352
	Hungary	641	102	260	176	262
	Norway	602	152	181	137	254
	Slovenia	603	200	210	143	284
	Sweden	630	153	184	130	343
	UK	620	133	219	142	325
	US	604	174	203	168	282
	Japan	620	103	258	189	270
			Fathers			
Married couple with youngest childe aged 0–6	Belgium	633	287	107	51	361
	Estonia	630	299	96	50	365
	Finland	607	339	100	63	331
	France	688	329	99	40	284
	Germany	618	305	105	59	353
	Hungary	636	321	83	71	329
	Norway	581	321	107	73	356
	Slovenia	601	369	81	56	334
	Sweden	597	318	122	67	336
	UK	600	373	92	60	315
	US	572	435	98	70	260
	Japan	605	517	27	33	259

Source: European countries (1998 - 2002); Harmonised European Time Use Surveys (European Communities); Japan (2006); Survey on Time Use and Leisure Activities (Ministry of Internal Affairs and Communications); US (2003); American Time Use Survey (U.S. Bureau of Labour Statistics).

are limited to those with children aged 0 to 5. Activities are divided into the following five categories: personal care, employment and related travel, domestic work, childcare, leisure, study and others. The time taken up by these activities adds up to 1440 minutes (24 hours) per day.[2]

In Japan's case, while no major differences were observed between the male and female partners in the couples in time used concerning "personal care" and "leisure, study and others," this was not the case with "employment and related travel," "domestic work" and "childcare." Compared with mothers, fathers devoted five times more time to employment and related travel (517 minutes versus 103), whereas fathers' involvement in domestic work paled besides that of mothers (27 minutes versus 258). The differential was also large in childcare, where fathers spent 33 minutes versus the 189 minutes spent by mothers in this activity.

Placing these figures in a comparative context, we find that only German and Hungarian mothers spent less time in employment and related travel than their Japanese counterparts. Japanese mothers spent more time on housework than mothers in all other countries except Hungary, while they topped the twelve-country list for time spent in childcare. Among the countries included in the comparison, Japanese fathers invested most time in employment and related travel, but they devoted the least time on domestic work; childcare; and leisure, study and others. Hence, by observing daily time use patterns, we find that among the twelve countries examined gender-based segregation of activities was most salient in Japan.

Changes in Time Spent on Childcare for Mothers and Fathers

Next we take a look at changes in time spent on childcare by individuals in households with children in Japan. Table 6.11 shows daily time use for households consisting of a married couple and at least one child under the age of 6. From this we can see that over time both sexes had been directing more time towards childcare. Mothers had increased their involvement in this category by 41 minutes and fathers by 23 minutes. Despite the increase in fathers' involvement in childcare, the larger increase on the part of mothers had resulted in the male–female differential growing from 137 minutes in 1986 to 155 minutes in 2006.

In contrast to childcare, mothers' involvement in domestic work and fathers' engagement in employment both saw a decrease, the former shrinking by 46 minutes (from 302 minutes in 1986 to 256 minutes in 2006), and the latter diminishing by 29 minutes (from 542 minutes in 1986 to 513 minutes in 2006). Following from the trend towards increased participation by fathers in both domestic work and childcare, the male–female differential for participation in unpaid work had shrunk from 428 minutes in 1986 (when mothers participated for 448 minutes and fathers for 20 minutes) to 385minutes in 2006 (when mothers participated for 443 minutes and fathers for 58 minutes).

Table 6.11 Trends in Daily Time Use by Mothers and Fathers with at Least One Child Under the Age of 6 (1986–2006)

	Sleep, personal care and meals	Employment and related travel	Housework, shopping and elderly care	Child care	Leisure, study and other
Mothers					
1986	608	122	302	146	260
1991	601	109	300	162	266
1996	617	92	292	159	279
2001	615	88	275	180	282
2006	621	109	256	187	265
Fathers					
1986	602	542	11	9	277
1996	604	508	20	17	291
2001	601	512	23	25	277
2006	607	513	26	32	260

Note: 1991 data for fathers could not be retrieved.

Changes in Time Spent on Childcare for Different Household Types

In this section we examine how time used in childcare had changed over time according to type of household. The two types we distinguish between are two-generation and three-generation households (where parents and children co-reside with one or more grandparent). Figure 6.1, which is based on data from the STULA surveys, shows how the relative share of these household types had changed between 1986 and 2006.[3] Simply put, households consisting only of parents and children had increased (from 74.8 per cent in 1986 to 87.7 per cent in 2006) while three-generation households had seen a substantial decrease (from 25.2 per cent to 12.3 per cent). This trend is borne out by other surveys as well, and it applies to the whole of Japan. For example, the percentage of three-generation households with children aged under 18 years was 27 per cent in 1986 but only 21.3 per cent in 2006 (Ministry of Health, Labour and Welfare (MHLW) 1986; 2006).

Table 6.12 shows time use data for fathers[4] of families with children under the age of 6 according to family type between 1986 and 2006. The data show no significant difference in time spent in childcare between fathers in two-generation and three-generation households. Those in the former spent a mere two to five minutes more taking care of children than those in the latter. No noteable difference between fathers in these two types of families appeared even if we consider changes over time. There were nevertheless disparities in the distribution of time use between these two groups: compared with two-generation families, fathers in three-generation households

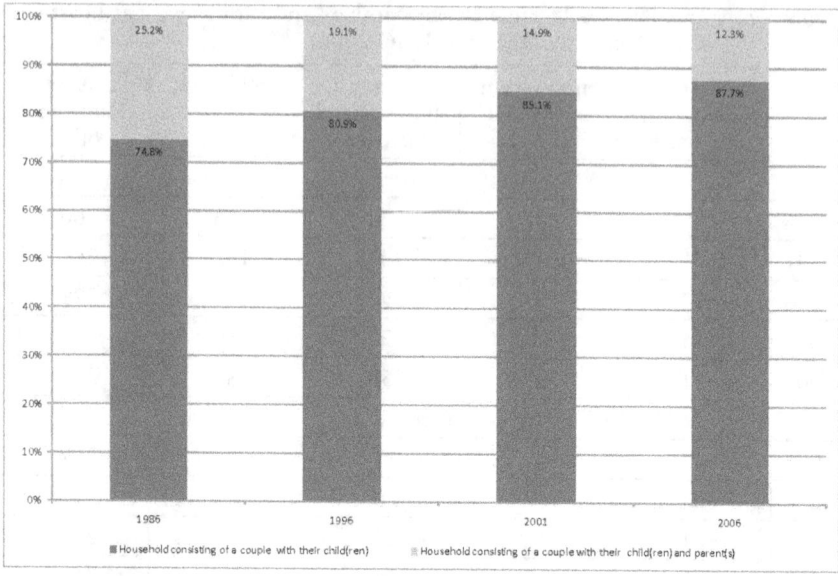

Figure 6.1 Changes in the relative share of two-generation and three-generation households with children under the age of six between 1986 and 2006.

enjoyed more personal care and leisure, study and other time even as they spent less time on childcare, domestic work and paid work.

Table 6.13 describes in similar fashion the time used by mothers[5] in childcare between 1986 and 2006 according to type of household. Compared to their peers in two-generation households, mothers in three-generation households had spent approximately 20 minutes less involved with childcare over this period. As for time spent in paid work, mothers in three-generation households had spent more time working than mothers living with their husband and children only, but this gap has been shrinking (with the former worked from 184 minutes to 154 minutes and the latter from 86 to 103).

Changes in Time Spent on Childcare by Mother's Employment Status

Next, we examine changes in time spent in childcare by mothers according not only to type of household but also labour force participation. To this end, Figure 6.2 illustrates how the employment rate of mothers had changed according to type of household using STULA data. While the overall female rate of employment had decreased between 1986 and 1996, it had increased thereafter. The employment rate for mothers in three-generation households had been higher (by between 18 to 25 percentage points) than that for mothers living with only the husband and children throughout the observed period, but this difference had been shrinking. Almost all of these trends had also been detected by other surveys.

Table 6.12 Time Use Distribution of Fathers in Families with at Least One Child Below 6 Years of Age by Type of Household (1986–2006)

	Sleep, personal care and meals	Employment and related travel	Housework, shopping and elderly care	Child care	Leisure, study and other
			Total		
1986	602	542	11	9	277
1996	604	508	20	17	291
2001	601	512	23	25	277
2006	607	513	26	32	260
		Fathers in two generation households: Couples with child(ren)			
1986	599	542	12	9	278
1996	601	510	20	18	292
2001	601	514	23	25	278
2006	605	517	27	33	259
		Fathers in three generation households: Couples with child(ren) and grandparents			
1986	611	537	9	7	275
1996	612	503	18	15	290
2001	611	501	19	22	289
2006	623	498	23	27	270

Note: 1991 data for fathers could not be retrieved.

Table 6.14 demonstrates how the time use of mothers with at least one child under the age of 6 had changed according to type of household and employment (two-generation vis-à-vis three-generation households, employed vis-à-vis non-employed mothers). We can see from this that time spent on childcare had increased across all of these types apart from 1996. From 1986 to 2001, it was non-employed mothers in three-generation households who spent most time in childcare, but in 2006 they were overtaken by non-employed mothers in two-generation families. No significant differences in time spent on childcare had been observed between employed mothers according to type of family (with the exception of 1996 when 100 minutes were spent by mothers in two-generation households against 79 minutes by mothers in three-generation households). Looking at overall time use, non-employed mothers spent relatively more time on childcare, domestic work and leisure and related activities than their employed peers, regardless of family type.

Let us summarise the findings regarding the influence of family type and employment status on time spent on childcare. First, for both mothers and fathers, we observed a trend towards an increase in childcare participation

Table 6.13 Time Use Distribution of Mothers in Families with at Least One Child Under the Age 6 by Type of Household (1986–2006)

	Sleep, personal care and meals	Employment and related travel	Housework, shopping and elderly care	Child care	Leisure, study and other
Total					
1986	608	122	302	146	260
1991	601	109	300	162	266
1996	617	92	292	159	279
2001	615	88	275	180	282
2006	621	109	256	187	265
Mothers in two generation households: Couples with child(ren)					
1986	610	95	311	149	276
1991	602	86	306	167	277
1996	616	77	295	163	289
2001	614	80	278	183	285
2006	620	103	258	189	270
Mothers in three generation households: Couples with child(ren) and grandparents					
1986	606	204	274	141	214
1991	606	184	281	145	225
1996	621	157	279	140	241
2001	620	135	262	167	257
2006	625	154	245	172	246

regardless of family type and labour force participation. However, fathers in three-generation households were distinctive in that they put less time into childcare, domestic work and paid work while directing more time towards personal care and leisure, study and others. In contrast, fathers living only with their wife and children spent more time on work and childcare as well as domestic work. It is possible that the co-residing grandparents in three-generation households shouldered some of the childcare and domestic work, allowing the father to use less time on these activities and more on personal care and leisure, study and others.

As for mothers, compared to those in two-generation households, those who co-reside with one or more grandparents spent more time working and less time doing housework. In the case of employed mothers, there was almost no difference in time spent on childcare observed across different household compositions, which suggests that a three-generation family provided little assistance from grandparents for childcare. However,

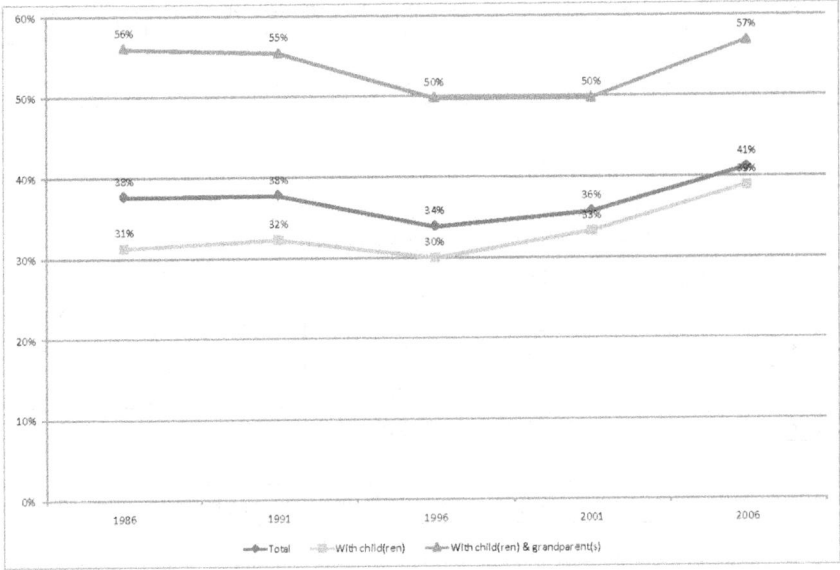

Figure 6.2 Labour force participation of mothers with at least one child under the age of 6 by type of household (1986–2006).

non-employed mothers living in three-generation households spent comparatively more time on housework and childcare activities (with time spent on childcare in 2006 presenting an exception). We inferred that mothers in three-generation households spent more time in paid work since the co-residing grandparents took responsibility for part of the unpaid domestic work where mothers were employed. Where mothers residing in three-generation households were non-employed, they may have performed unpaid work on behalf of the whole family (including the potentially frail grandparents' share), leading to more time spent on unpaid work as their husbands contributed relatively little time towards childcare.

Childcare Participation by Single and Married Mothers in Two-generation Households

This section examines the characteristics of time spent on childcare in the case of single mothers with at least one child younger than 6 years of age. Figure 6.3 traces changes in the labour force participation rate of these single mothers based on data from the STULA. Compared to married mothers residing with their husband and children (see Figure 6.2), a considerably higher number of single mothers had taken part in paid employment.

Table 6.15 shows the daily time use distribution of single mothers. For those who were employed, we see that over time, relatively less time had

Table 6.14 Time Use Distribution of Mothers with One or More Children Under the Age of 6 According to HouseholdType and Employment Status (1986–2006)

	Sleep, personal care and meals	Employment and related travel	Housework, shopping and elderly care	Child care	Leisure, study and other
Total					
Employed					
1986	602	318	229	84	206
1991	596	283	243	99	220
1996	612	268	232	94	233
2001	611	244	225	112	250
2006	618	260	208	128	224
Not employed					
1986	612	4	345	185	294
1991	606	2	337	200	295
1996	619	1	323	192	304
2001	617	2	303	218	299
2006	622	1	291	230	295
Mothers in two generation households: Couples with child(ren)					
Employed					
1986	603	293	237	84	221
1991	591	261	252	102	236
1996	609	253	237	100	241
2001	612	237	228	112	252
2006	618	259	209	128	228
Not employed					
1986	612	4	344	179	301
1991	606	1	334	198	300
1996	619	1	320	190	307
2001	615	2	302	218	302
2006	622	1	290	230	299
Mothers in three generation households: Couples with child(ren) and grandparent(s)					
Employed					
1986	602	365	213	85	180
1991	602	327	227	92	191
1996	621	309	220	79	211
2001	611	273	212	112	233
2006	623	265	205	129	218

continued

Table 6.14 continued

	Not employed				
1986	611	8	350	212	259
1991	610	4	372	212	263
1996	620	4	339	202	275
2001	629	1	310	222	277
2006	627	2	299	227	284

been spent in paid work and domestic work while more time had been spent on childcare. This was a trend that was also to be seen in the case of employed married mothers. In comparison with them, however, single mothers had significantly longer work hours and spent significantly less time on childcare. Even non-employed single mothers invested less time in childcare than their married peers. However, this result should be treated with caution due to the low number of non-employed single mothers in the sample.

The Results in Relation to Childcare Policy

We have seen that there was a trend towards more time being invested in childcare by both mothers and fathers. We found also that work time had been decreasing for both sexes; that fathers had slightly been increasing their involvement in domestic work; and that mothers had been spending

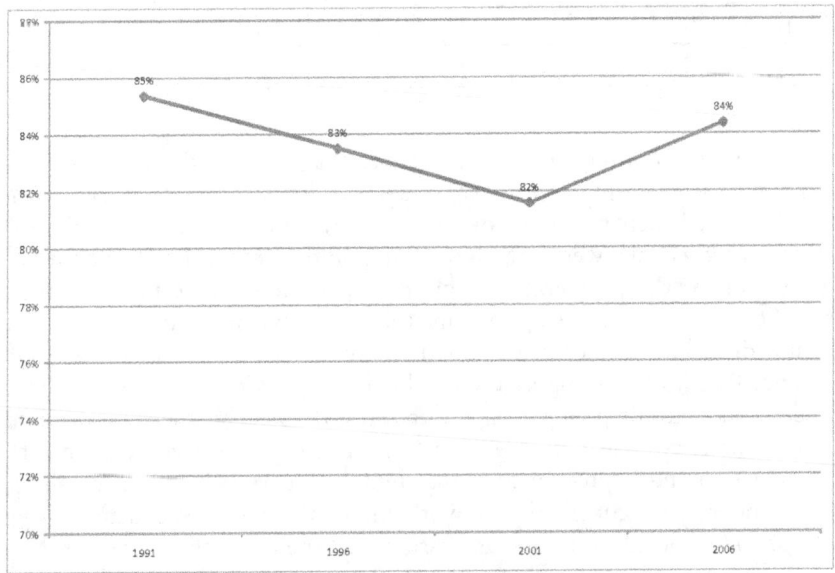

Figure 6.3 Changes in the labour force participation rate of single mothers with at least one child under the age of 6 (1991–2006).

Table 6.15 Time Use Data for Single Mothers with at Least One Child Under the Age of 6 by Type of Employment (1986–2006)

	Sleep, personal care and meals	Employment and related travel	Housework, shopping and elderly care	Child care	Leisure, study and other
Total					
1986	624	292	199	58	266
1991	620	311	198	68	241
1996	635	288	180	60	276
2001	633	287	175	84	262
2006	620	295	184	101	242
Employed					
1986	613	377	171	43	234
1991	615	363	177	47	239
1996	637	342	171	37	255
2001	626	355	156	58	247
2006	614	349	158	88	230
Not employed					
1986	662	6	197	104	373
1991	665	0	305	169	301
1996	625	0	232	179	404
2001	664	0	248	194	334
2006	651	1	291	181	317

significantly less time on domestic tasks than previously. Furthermore, examining time spent on childcare in detail, we discovered that while men had increased their participation by just a few minutes, mothers—regardless of whether they were employed or not, and whether they lived in two-generation or three-generation households, or were single mothers—had significantly been increasing the time they spent caring for children.

It is difficult to demonstrate how these trends and childcare policies were related. Policies that support the combination of work and childcare have underpinned family policy in Japan since the 1990s. The major means used for this objective had been the improvement of child-care services, and the introduction and improvement of the child-care leave system. Since policies that support the reconciliation of work and family had been enacted during the period of observation, it was possible that the increase in time spent on childcare by working mothers was partially due to such policies. However, if we consider that *non*-employed mothers were also spending more time on childcare, it becomes harder to argue that this was a trend prompted by family policy. Furthermore, it is puzzling that time spent on childcare should have decreased (regardless of family type or employment status) at a time when the number of children per household had been diminishing. Recalling that participation in housework had been decreasing, it may be that mothers were simply transferring the excess time gained towards childcare rather than being influenced by any family policy. Another possible explanation is that there was a tendency to assign higher importance to childcare than housekeeping. In addition, the fact that single mothers spent conspicuously less time on childcare compared to married mothers in two-generation households suggests that for this group the reconciliation of childcare and work still presented great difficulties.

Turning to the time spent on childcare and domestic work by fathers, a slight increase had been observed in both categories. It is possible that this trend had reflected the influence of gender equality policies that were, to some extent, reconfiguring the previously fixed gender-based division of labour as well as changes in values. Alternatively, it may have been the result of labour market policies, such as the increasing practice of allowing a two-day holiday from work per week and restrictions on long working hours. The increase in part-time jobs may have resulted in many mothers allocating more time towards childcare instead of to paid work.

TIME SPENT ON CARE FOR THE ELDERLY

In this section we consider long-term trends in the amount of time that Japanese men and women spend on caring for the elderly. First, we look at changes in time used daily in this activity. Next, we make use of a survey conducted after the implementation of Long-Term Care Insurance (LTCI) to investigate how time spent on caring is influenced by the use or non-use of caring assistance[6]. LTCI is a mandatory social insurance programme for elderly care. It was introduced in 2000 in response to increasing life expectancy, smaller household size and women's increasing rates of labour force participation, which meant that taking care of elderly within the family had become increasingly difficult. LTCI encourages home care services rather than institutional services. Thus whereas the monthly number of users of at home care services rapidly increased over seven years (1,236,000 in 2000, to 2,625,000 in 2007), the users of institutional services rose more moderately (604,000 in 2000 to 819,000 in 2007; MHLW 2007).

Figure 6.4 draws on STULA to highlight the share of men and women who are usually caring for an elderly family member.[7] Against a background of progressive demographic ageing, we observe slight increases in the share of those who provided care within the family. For each year that data were available, a larger percentage of women than men spent time for the elderly.

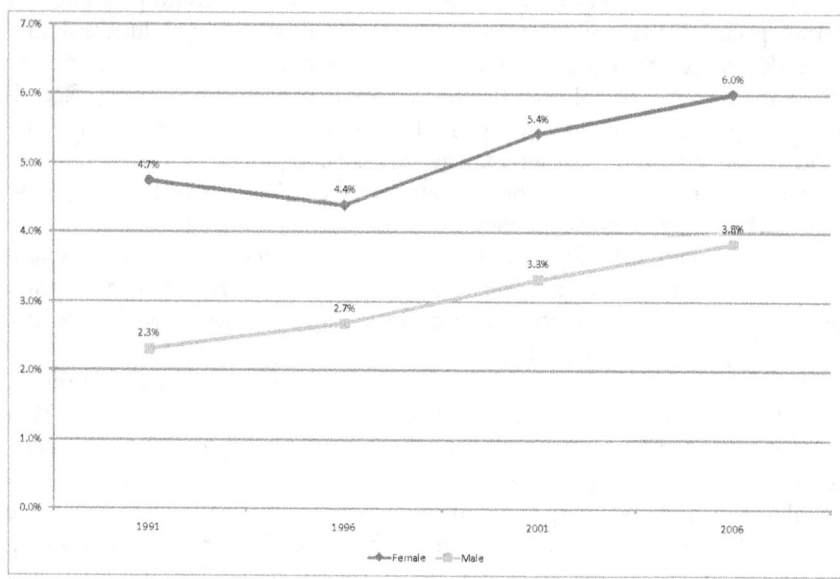

Figure 6.4 Percentage of men and women who usually care for a family member (1991–2006).

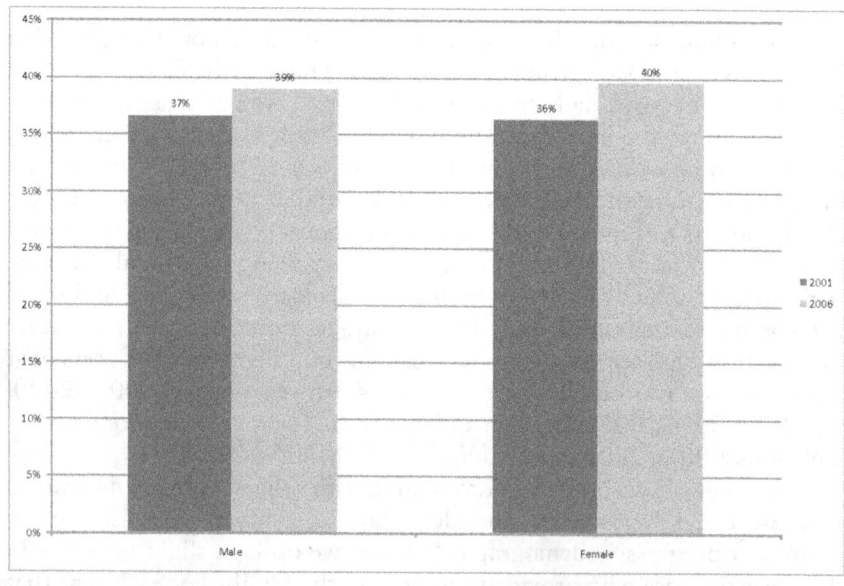

Figure 6.5 Percentage of people caring for family members living in separate residence (2001–2006).

Respondents who are caring for family members are classified into those who provide care at home and those who provide care outside the home. The latter are those who care for their parents or parents-in-law living in separate residences. Figure 6.5 shows the proportion of people providing care outside the home in 2001 and 2006 by sex. In 2006, the percentage of those providing care outside the home increased for both males and females. Note that, while care outside the home increased, more than 60 per cent of males and females were providing care at home.

Table 6.16 gives a five-category breakdown of daily time use for men and women who provide family-based care for the elderly. We see that the amount of time women spent on caring had in fact decreased between 1991 and 2006, from 72 to 60 minutes. A major downward trend—from 73 to 62 minutes—was observed between 1996 and 2001 in particular. At the same time, men's participation in care had increased over the examined period, albeit only very slightly.

The Influence of Caring Assistance on Time Spent on Care

Let us now look at how the use or non-use of caring assistance influences the amount of time spent on care by women and men. Figure 6.6 shows how large a share of those who provide family-based care also use caring assistance. Overall, the share of assistance users had increased between 2001 and 2006. For both of these time points, a higher share of men than women made use of caring assistance.

Table 6.16 The Daily Time Use Distribution of Men and Women Who Provide Care for a Family Member (1991–2006)

	Sleep, personal care and meals	Employment and related travel	Housework, shopping and child care	Elderly care	Leisure, study and other
Female					
1991	623	179	257	72	310
1996	634	158	254	73	320
2001	628	149	252	62	348
2006	621	151	266	60	341
Male					
1991	622	392	41	29	356
1996	642	357	42	30	369
2001	634	327	50	29	400
2006	638	308	62	31	403

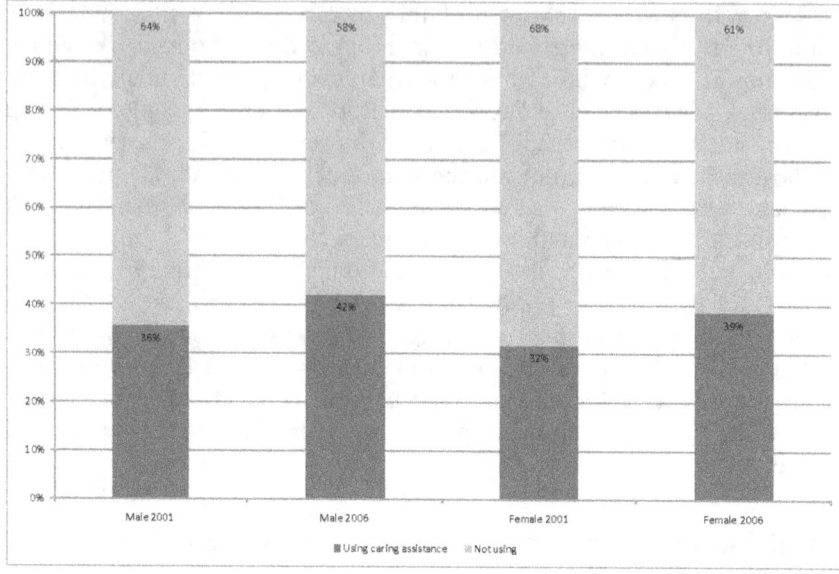

Figure 6.6 Percentage of caregivers for family members 65 years old and over using caring assistance.

Table 6.17 highlights differences in caring time between caring assistance users and non-users. For both women and men, those who also used caring assistance appeared to spend more time on care than those who did not use such assistance. It is likely that this was due to the higher care needs of the elderly who were being cared for by both family members *and* professional care workers. If we compare how much time women used on caring in 2001 and 2006, we find a marked decrease for those who were making use of caring assistance (from 85 to 76 minutes).

The Influence of Elderly Care Policies on Time Use

One of the objectives of the LTCI was the alleviation of the care burden on families via the provision of external (non-family) care services. The LTCI was established against a context of rapid ageing, increasing life expectancy and an attendant increase in the care needs of the elderly. In addition, the heavy care burden shouldered by elderly wives caring for their elderly husbands (and vice versa) and daughters-in-law furnishing care for their husband's parents was viewed as a pressing concern prior to the enactment of the new insurance plan. This heavy burden that fell primarily on female caregivers reflected the strength of gender norms and role segregation that prescribed caring as primarily a women's responsibility—one that surpassed even childcare in relative importance. Thus females accounted for 76.4 per cent of main caregivers in 2001 and 71.9 per cent in 2007 (MHLW 2001; 2007).

Table 6.17 The Daily Time Use Distribution of Women and Men who Provide Care to an Elderly Family Member (or Members) According to the Use of Caring Assistance

	Year	Sleep, personal care and meals	Employment and related travel	Housework, shopping and child care	Elderly care	Other
		Female				
Using caring assistance	2001	626	145	248	85	335
Using caring assistance	2006	629	137	267	76	331
Not using caring assistance	2001	629	151	256	54	353
Not using caring assistance	2006	619	158	265	53	346
		Male				
Using caring assistance	2001	634	308	55	38	403
Using caring assistance	2006	642	283	70	42	404
Not using caring assistance	2001	635	335	47	25	396
Not using caring assistance	2006	637	319	58	26	400

The data on daily time use in the period following the introduction of the LTCI suggest that the scheme has had differing effects for men and women. It is entirely possible that the decrease in women's care provision observed between 1996 and 2001 was due to the introduction of the new insurance system. Crucially, when disaggregating the newer survey data into caring assistance users and non-users, we found that the former spent significantly less time on elderly care in 2001 than they did in 2006. Men, on the other hand, had slightly increased their involvement in care, with users of caring assistance spending four minutes longer on care in 2006 compared to 2001.

DISCUSSION

In this chapter, we presented an analysis of the time allocated to care by Japanese males and females, its determining factors and its change over time, by the operations of time use surveys.

Firstly, according to the analysis conducted in the first half of this chapter, the time spent on paid and unpaid work was distinctly different between males and females. Males spent longer time on paid work than females, and females spent longer time on unpaid care work than males, which held true even after controlling for the respective attributes of males and females.

The result of a regression analysis on unpaid care work and care of persons by males and females was that two demographic variables, marital status and co-residence with children under 6 years of age, strongly affected the time spent on unpaid care work and care of persons in the case of females. As for socio-economic variables, while a higher educational standard lengthened the time spent on these in the case of females, no effect was observed with variation in household income. In the case of males, while no effect was observed with variation in marital status, time spent on unpaid care work became shorter when the individual co-resides with an elderly person aged 65 years or over, and the care of persons became longer with children under 6 years of age. As for socio-economic variables, while unpaid care work became longer with a higher male educational standard, unpaid care work decreased as household income increased.

Secondly, in the second half of the chapter, where time spent on childcare and care for the elderly were examined using time series data, we first recognised the tendency that time spent on childcare was increasing, regardless of sex, household composition (whether two-generation households comprising only of a married couple, three-generation households or single mother households) and employment status. A similar tendency toward longer time spent on childcare is also recognised in other developed countries. While the employment rate of females is increasing and the number of children per household is decreasing, particularly in western countries, which might be expected to result in less time spent on childcare, it is pointed out that in fact this is increasing for both males and females (Gershuny 2000, Bianchi 2000, Gauthier, Smeeding and Furstenberg 2004, Sayer, Bianchi and Robinson 2004).

Why is time spent on childcare increasing? The regression analysis in which we analyze the determining factors of time spent on childcare by using micro data of the 2001 survey (Table 6.9) reveals that time spent on childcare became longer for both males and females who were highly educated. While higher education lengthened time spent on childcare, no significant effect was observed with variation in household income. From the results concerning higher education and household income, we can consider that time spent on childcare has increased as a result of the development of a "highly-educated person's view of child rearing," that is, a great deal of time and care is devoted to the upbringing of children regardless of one's economic resources, not that higher education lengthens the time spent on childcare because of an increase in one's economic resources. Also, as for factors regarding the children themselves, the age of the youngest child, not the number of children, seems to be the main factor affecting time spent on childcare. In addition, it is found that time spent on childcare decreased with employment, being a single mother, or with the increase in the number of household members other than children.

Finally, in respect of time spent on care for the elderly, following the introduction of the LTCI in 2000, the participation rate in elderly care increased for both males and females and the time spent on care decreased for females and slightly increased for males.[8] This is especially the case among those who use nursing care assistance services. From this, we can consider that the LTCI has had the effect of reducing the burden of elderly care on females, while increasing male commitment to elderly care.

NOTES

1. These data were anonymously processed micro data provided by the Research Centre for Information and Statistics of Social Science, Institute of Economic Research, Hitotsubashi University. The micro data of STULA surveys conducted in 2001 were provided by the centre.
2. Due to rounding errors resulting from the re-coding of international data into the above five categories, there are cases where the total time spent on the activities amounts to slightly more or less than 1440 minutes.
3. These data do not specify whether it is the parents of the husband, or of the wife who are co-residing in the family dwelling.
4. "Father" means the father of children, not a grandfather in a three-generation household.
5. "Mother" means the mother of children, not a grandmother in a three-generation household.
6. In this paper, "caring assistance" means not only care services by the LTCI but also care services outside the LTCI. The two can not be distinguished in the STULA.
7. STULA classified respondents according to whether they usually care for their family members or not. A person who usually provides care is further classified according to the person/people for whom he/she is caring for and where he/she is providing the care. The classification is thus as follow for those usually providing care:

    Usually providing care
    - Care provision for family members 65 years old and over
    Providing care at home/care provided outside the home
    - Care provision for family members under 65 years old
    Providing care at home/Caring provided outside the home
    "Care" refers to helping a person to have a meal, take a bath, dress, move, or carry out other daily movements. "Care" also includes care for people who have not been recognised as persons who require care under the LCTI. Caring for persons who are temporarily sick is excluded.
8. Regression analysis could not be conducted for time spent on nursing care due to the shortage of actors.

REFERENCES

Bianchi, Suzanne M. 2000. "Maternal employment and time with children: Dramatic change or surprising continuity?" *Demography*, Vol. 37, No. 4, pp. 401–414.

Gauthier, Anne H, Timothy M. Smeeding, and Frank F. Furstenberg Jr. 2004. "Are parents investing less time in children? Trends in selected industrialized countries", *Population & Development Review*, Vol 30, No. 4, pp. 647–672.

Gershuny, Jonathan. 2000. *Changing Times: Work and Leisure in Postindustrial Society*. Oxford University Press, Oxford.

Ministry of Health, Labour and Welfare (MHLW). 1986. *Compreensive Survey of Living Conditions of the People on Health and Welfare* (Kokumin Seikatsu Kiso Chōsa), Tokyo.

Ministry of Health, Labour and Welfare (MHLW). 2001. *Compreensive Survey of Living Conditions of the People on Health and Welfare* (Kokumin Seikatsu Kiso Chōsa), Tokyo.

Ministry of Health, Labour and Welfare (MHLW). 2006. *Compreensive Survey of Living Conditions of the People on Health and Welfare* (Kokumin Seikatsu Kiso Chōsa), Tokyo.

Ministry of Health, Labour and Welfare (MHLW). 2007. *Compreensive Survey of Living Conditions of the People on Health and Welfare* (Kokumin Seikatsu Kiso Chōsa), Tokyo.

Ministry of Health, Labour and Welfare (MHLW). 2007. *Report on Long-term Care Insurance Service* (Kaigo Hoken Jigyo Jyokyo Chōsa), Tokyo.

Ministry of Internal Affairs and Communications. 1986. *Survey on Time Use and Leisure Activities* (Shakai Seikatsu Kihon Chōsa), Tokyo.

Ministry of Internal Affairs and Communications. 1991. *Survey on Time Use and Leisure Activities* (Shakai Seikatsu Kihon Chōsa), Tokyo.

Ministry of Internal Affairs and Communications. 1996. *Survey on Time Use and Leisure Activities* (Shakai Seikatsu Kihon Chōsa), Tokyo.

Ministry of Internal Affairs and Communications. 2001. *Survey on Time Use and Leisure Activities* (Shakai Seikatsu Kihon Chōsa), Tokyo.

Ministry of Internal Affairs and Communications. 2006. *Survey on Time Use and Leisure Activities* (Shakai Seikatsu Kihon Chōsa).

Sayer, Liana, Suzanne M. Bianchi and John P. Robinson. 2004. "Are parents investing less in children? Trends in mothers' and fathers' time with children" *American Journal of Sociology*, Vol. 110, No. 1, pp. 1–43.

7 The Case of Nicaragua

Isolda Espinosa González

INTRODUCTION

What do we know about how Nicaraguans use time and, in particular, the time they devote to care? If responding to this question is important under any welfare and care regime, it is especially important when there are market and state "failures" in meeting the basic needs of the population. In this context, one would expect a much larger part of the unpaid work to be done in households and communities.

From the very inception of economics as a discipline, the central corpus of its work has been developed with a view to understanding capitalist production (Hausman 1984, and Albelda 1997, cited in Carrasco 2006). Thus, "work" has been defined to include only those activities that are actual or potential objects of commerce. This concept of work has profoundly affected the recognition of women's contribution to the economy and to the society.

Feminist economics regards this approach as incomplete, since a society's survival depends not only on its pattern of economic production, but also on the pattern of social reproduction,1 which includes unpaid service production for household's consumption. Under prevailing theoretical approaches, the invisibility of reproductive work has also rendered reproductive work—and those who perform it—socially invisible. More specifically, what is obscured is the relationship between production and reproduction characteristics of the capitalist system (Picchio 1994).

For feminist economics, social reproduction requires a set of activities generally designated as work, most of which fall outside what is typically defined as being part of "the economy." The most important of these activities, in terms of both content and time consumed, are (unpaid) domestic work and caregiving (Carrasco 2006).

Historically, care work has been provided by women within the household on an unpaid basis. However, it may be supplemented by paid work performed in the home, paid work in the public or private service sectors, and volunteer work. According to Picchio (1999), however, the ultimate responsibility for reconciling these forms of work, and for dealing with their less-than-sufficient yield, continues to be borne by those who perform unpaid work within the family—especially women.

172 *Isolda Espinosa González*

To address care work in Nicaragua, this chapter (a) categorises work-care regimes in Nicaragua according to the different ways in which households combine activity in the labour market with unpaid care work, and the manner in which they allocate these activities among their members; and (b) estimates the contribution to the national economy made by women's unpaid care work, in order to reveal this hidden cost of economic production. To this end, we have analysed data from the time use section of the 1998 National Standard of Living Survey (Encuesta Nacional de Medición del Nivel de Vida, or EMNV) conducted by Nicaragua's National Institute of Statistics and Census (Instituto Nacional de Estadísticas y Censos, or INEC).

The study sample, which is representative of the national population, comprises 8,756 persons of 6 years of age or older who were regular residents of the 2,325 selected housing units surveyed between April and August for the time use section of the 1998 EMNV. Each of these individuals was asked twenty-five questions, in order to establish whether he or she had carried out specified activities the *day prior* to the interview. The time spent in various daily activities was also checked, ensuring that they totalled 24 hours. The population's socio-demographic and economic characteristics were registered on other sections of the 1998 EMNV.

Obtaining information on time use by asking about pre-defined activities is problematic inasmuch as activities not covered by the questions (e.g. care of older adults) may be inadvertently omitted. In addition, the reliance on respondents' memory increases the chance that responses will reflect what respondents "normally" do (or think they should do), rather than what they actually did on the reference day. Basing the reports on respondents' memory also affects the quality of the data on the time devoted to different activities, since respondents have a tendency to round off times.

Furthermore, the fact that the number of questions related to different activities was not constant may have affected the final time use data. For example, there were four questions on household work, but only one on childcare. (In the latter case, no details were solicited regarding the specific activities involved, or to determine whether the children cared for were members of the household, as opposed to members of other households.) Responses thus reflected only what the respondents themselves considered to be childcare and their subjective perceptions of time.

Despite these limitations, and as shown in the chapter more broadly, the data collected through the survey are valid and extremely useful, not only for assessing actual time use in Nicaragua, but for public policy-making that would hopefully deal with the many tensions involved in balancing paid work and unpaid care work.

WHAT DO WE MEAN BY WORK AND CARE WORK?

There are two basic definitions that are important for this study: employment-related "work" and unpaid care work. The definition of employment-related work used by the Nicaraguan government is based on the standards and guidelines of the System of National Accounts (SNA). The labour force statistics consider as employed those persons doing productive activities within the SNA production boundary. The SNA, however, excludes unpaid domestic and personal services performed by households for their own consumption, such as food preparation; care, education and training of children; care of the ill and the elderly; and cleaning, maintenance and repair of durable goods, etc. (See Chapter 1).

The present study adopted a modified version of the SNA definition of work. Collection of water and wood, which in the SNA are part of employment-related work, are excluded here on account of the fact that they are not considered as such in the official statistics of Nicaragua. They are therefore included here as part of unpaid care work. In effect, SNA work covers the following categories:

- Paid work
- Unpaid work in family or non-family firms or businesses[2]

Care work, on the other hand, is defined as activities, whether paid or not, which are done for the household-family with the aim of assuring the daily reproduction of its members. Unpaid care work is similar, but excludes any care work that is paid.

In view of its objectives, the present study examines only *unpaid care work*. Based on the content of the time use section of the 1998 EMNV, the activities included are classified in two categories:

- Domestic tasks, including cooking, housecleaning, dishwashing and laundry, ironing, house repairs, household shopping and collection of fuel and water
- Care for persons, including childcare and care of the ill. (Adult care more generally is not under examination here). However, the way in which the questions in the time use section of the 1998 EMNV were formulated makes it impossible to determine whether the persons being cared for did or did not belong to the interviewees' households

We decided not to include community and related services on account of the fact that, because of the way in which the questions were asked, it is not possible to determine to which category of the SNA they correspond.

WHAT IS THE SOCIO-DEMOGRAPHIC AND ECONOMIC PROFILE OF THE STUDY POPULATION?

To study the time use patterns of Nicaraguans, we use a combination of variables, among which sex is the central axis of the analysis given the importance of gender roles for time use. In this section we discuss what the surveyed population looks like in terms of these variables. Based on this depiction we can tell whether the sample is reliable in respect of the population as a whole and better understand the primary results concerning time use.

The sample is almost equally distributed between the sexes: 49.7 per cent men and 50.3 women. Just over half of the participants in the sample (52.6 per cent) lived in urban areas. However, disaggregation by sex shows the men are almost equally distributed between urban and rural areas, while a significant majority of the women reside in urban areas (55.6 per cent).

The greater propensity of rural women to migrate to cities reflects the greater job opportunities available in urban centres, where these women traditionally find work as domestic employees or, more recently, in *maquila* enterprises in free zones.

The age groups used to analyse the information are based on a combination of the official Nicaraguan definition of childhood (0 to 17) and of women's reproductive age (15 to 49). Although the behaviour of the retirement-age population (65+) is also of interest, it was necessary to aggregate this group with the 50–64 year group, since the number of observations in the 65+ population constituted less than 5 per cent of the total population interviewed.

The sample was concentrated in the first two age groups, with the 18–49 group predominating, especially among women. Thus, slightly less than half of the population interviewed consisted of individuals in the peak productive and reproductive age group. The sample in the 50+ group was evenly divided between the sexes, and thus does not reflect women's greater life expectancy.

As to age distribution within the sample, 64.1 per cent of the sample (63.3 per cent of males and 64.9 per cent of females) fell in the 15- to 64-year-old group.

We categorised individuals according to whether they were members of conjugal unions (whether married or not[3]) at the time of the interview, had been in the past (i.e. were currently separated, divorced or widowed) or never had been (single people). Using this categorisation, slightly under half of the population aged 12 years or older was married or in conjugal unions, and over one third was single. Men and women were more or less equally likely to be married or in conjugal unions. Interestingly, the proportion of single men is 12 percentage points higher than that of single women. The percentage of separated, divorced or widowed men is approximately one third the percentage of separated/divorced/widowed women. In other words, men who have had a stable couple relationship that ends are unlikely to continue living without a partner.

In Nicaragua, information on conjugal status is sought on individuals 12 years old and older, as a result of the early average age at which women enter a first union.[4] However, inclusion of the population aged 15 and younger affects the data on conjugal status, increasing the relative weight of single persons and reducing that of the other categories. Thus, for example, more than half of the 15+ population is married or in conjugal unions—7 percentage points higher than for the broader age group. Conversely, the proportion of single people is nearly 9 points lower.

Respondents were categorised according to the type of household to which they belonged. The categorisation was based on the stage of the household members' life cycle. Three groups were defined: children (under 18), adults (18–64) and older adults (65 and over). The various possible combinations of these groups produced seven types of households: adults and children; children, adults and older adults; adults only; adults and older adults; only older adults; older adults and children; and children only. However, the last four types combined represent a mere 3.1 per cent of the total. Meanwhile, slightly over three quarters of the respondents belong to households composed of adults and children, without significant differences according to sex. The other household types to which respondents belong, in descending order of incidence among respondents, were as follows. A total of 16.3 per cent of respondents belong to three-generation households (children, adults and older adults), with women more likely than men to be members of such households. Adults-only households account for less than 5 per cent of respondents, and (unlike the previous group) men are more likely than women to belong to such households.

The presence of young children can have a substantial impact on the amount of unpaid care work done. Two fifths of the surveyed population live in households without children under 6 years. The rest are evenly divided between households with one such child and households with two or more. The distribution of women and men in the latter categories is the same.

In terms of economic activity, we utilise the categories used in traditional labour statistics, which are based on SNA definitions of production, and which consider persons who have performed some "work" during the previous week to be employed, those who have not worked, but have sought work, to be unemployed, and those who neither worked nor actively sought work to be economically inactive.

Nicaragua defines the working-age population as 10 to 64. However, the 1998 EMNV investigated the economic activity status of the population from age 6 and over, in order to investigate the extent of child labour in the country. As is customary, the calendar week prior to the interview was the reference period used. For the time use section of the survey, however, the reference period was the day prior to the interview. This discrepancy explains some apparent inconsistencies, such as the phenomenon of individuals who were unemployed (the previous week) performing paid work (the previous day).

One half of the population interviewed was economically inactive, and less than one half were employed, but there are significant differences by sex. A majority (60.8 per cent) of men were employed, and only one third were economically inactive, while less than one third of women were employed, and 67.3 per cent were economically inactive. The unemployed population constituted only 5.2 per cent of the total, with the proportion of men 1.3 percentage points higher than that of women.

In the 15- to 64-year-old population (i.e. the population capable of fully engaging in work), the proportion of employed individuals is 16.0 percentage points higher than for the broader age group, with a greater rise in the figure for men than for women (21.3 points and 11.2 points), while the economically inactive population drops by 17.7 points (the figure for men this time falling more than for women—23.1 points vs. 12.7 points).

For the purpose of the analysis, household monetary income was defined to include all monetary income of household members, whether from work, income from property, current transfers or extraordinary income from sources such as inheritances or insurance payments. The income ranges defining the quintiles are shown in the following paragraph.

As may be seen, quintile 1, which has an upper bound of C$410, includes some households without any monetary income during the calendar month prior to the interview. This is explained largely by the fact that the survey was conducted between April and August, before the harvest of annual and perennial crops—the time when households whose sole economic activity is agricultural receive the income from the sale of their products. The upper bounds for the remaining four quintiles are C$950, C$1,612, C$2,997 and C$140,333 respectively.

To understand what the preceding figures mean, we note that in 1998 the poverty line5 was C$355.00 per person, and the nation's average household size was 5.4 individuals. Thus, an average household required monthly monetary income of C$1,917.00 or more to cover its basic consumption needs and not be classified as poor.6 This means that the households in quintiles 1, 2 and 3 and some of those in quintile 4 do not have the necessary financial resources to cover their basic consumption needs.

This is no significant differences in the distribution of men and women by household income quintile. However, there is a very slightly greater tendency for women to live in households in quintiles 3 and 5.

In short, the preceding summary analysis confirms that the structure of the survey population matches that of the National Population Census of 1995 reflecting the main demographic and economic trends of the past decade.

WORK-CARE REGIMES OF THE 15 TO 64 YEAR OLD POPULATION

What are the time use patterns of the population aged 15–64 years? These are the ages which cover the peak of productive capacity as well as the reproductive years of women (15–49 years). In order to answer this question we analyse SNA work, and paid work in particular, together with unpaid care work. We subsequently deepen the study by looking at time spend on care of children.

To analyse the way in which the population distributed its time among the different activities in 1998, we use three basic indicators:

- Rate of participation, which shows the proportion of the population that undertakes the given activity, irrespective of the time spent on it
- Mean time per participant, which refers to the mean number of hours spent per day on the activity by those who undertake the activity
- Mean population time, which is a synthetic indicator based on the previous two, and is defined as the mean number of hours spent per day on the activity averaged over the full population

Because the first two indicators refer only to those who undertake the activity, neither of which on its own provides sufficient information on the time use of the full population, it is necessary to analyse them together.

In the following section we present three main findings: The distribution of men's and women's time by type of work and by basic socio-demographic and economic characteristics, and multivariate analysis to establish the strength of the relationship between unpaid care work and care of persons with a range of variables.

Distribution of Time Between the Main Types of Work

All the activities that a person does can be classified into three major categories according to the SNA: SNA work, unpaid care work (UCW) and personal care or non-productive activities (see Table 7.1).

There are big differences in the participation rates of men and women in SNA work and unpaid care work. In the first case, the participation rate of men is more than double that of women; in contrast, for UCW women show higher rates of participation. The difference in the rates for women and men are less for unpaid care work than for SNA work. This is probably due to the inclusion of collection of water and wood as part of unpaid care work, as these are activities that in some cases are done by adult men and/or boys.

The participation rates in non-productive activities are 100 per cent for both women and men, which confirms that all do at least one personal activity (sleeping, eating, bathing, etc).

In terms of the mean time spent on each of the three activity categories, for a particular sex the mean per actor will be bigger than the population mean. This difference increases with lower participation and vice versa. This is the reason that the difference (between the two means) for the mean time spent on SNA work is less for men than for women. In contrast, the gap for mean time spent on UCW is less for women than for men. In the

Table 7.1 Participation Rates, Mean Actor Time and Mean Population Time of the Population 15–64 Years by Sex and SNA Category

	Total	Male	Female
Participation rate (%)			
SNA	53.9	74.9	33.7
UCW	70.8	50.8	90.1
Non-productive activities	100.0	100.0	100.0
Mean actor time (hours per day)			
SNA	8.2	8.5	7.6
UCW	5.2	3.0	6.3
Non-productive activities	15.9	16.1	15.7
Mean population time (hours per day)			
SNA	4.4	6.4	2.6
UCW	3.6	1.5	5.7
Non-productive activities	15.9	16.1	15.7

case of non-productive activities the difference is zero, given that the participation rate is 100 per cent for both sexes.

We note that although only a third of women do SNA work, and the time that they spend on this work is only 10 per cent less than that of men. In other words, these women are subjected to tension in the use of time that does not face men.

According to Table 7.2, in terms of both total SNA work and each of its components, the participation of men is a little more than double the participation of women. The difference in the time devoted by participants to paid work is only 8 per cent, but with unpaid SNA work the difference increases to 39 per cent, both in favour of men. The difference increases to 145 per cent and 200 per cent, for paid SNA work and unpaid SNA work respectively, when we consider the mean population time.

With unpaid care work, women have higher participation rates and mean times than men (see Table 7.3). The biggest differences are observed for care of persons and domestic chores, for which the participation rate of women is more than 4 and 2 times respectively that of men. For both sexes, higher rates of participation are recorded for domestic chores.

If we look at actor means, the time spent by women in these same activities is 50 per cent and 100 per cent more than the corresponding times for men. In contrast, for collection of water and wood the differences are less stark. However, if we take the mean population time, the difference between the time spent by women and men for care of persons and domestic chores increases to 550 per cent and 460 per cent respectively.

Table 7.2 Participation Rates, Mean Actor Time and Mean Population Time of the Population 15–64 Years in SNA Work by Sex

	Total	Male	Female
Participation rate (%)			
SNA	53.9	74.9	33.7
Paid work	42.9	60.1	26.3
Unpaid work	9.7	12.9	6.6
Mean actor time (hours per day)			
SNA	8.2	8.5	7.6
Paid work	8.8	9.0	8.3
Unpaid work	6.4	7.1	5.1
Mean population time (hours per day)			
SNA	4.4	6.4	2.6
Paid work	3.8	5.4	2.2
Unpaid work	0.6	0.9	0.3

Table 7.3 Participation Rates, Mean Participant Time and Mean Population Time of the Population 15–64 Years in Unpaid Care Work by Sex

	Total	Male	Female
Participation rate (%)			
UCW	70.8	50.8	90.1
Care of persons	22.5	7.9	36.5
Household maintenance	62.0	35.9	87.1
Collection of fuel and water	25.5	23.5	27.5
Mean actor time (hours per day)			
SNA	5.2	3.0	6.3
Care of persons	2.9	2.1	3.0
Household maintenanc	4.1	2.5	4.8
Collection of fuel and wate	1.7	1.9	1.5
Mean population time (hours per day)			
SNA	3.6	1.5	5.7
Care of persons	0.6	0.2	1.1
Household maintenanc	2.6	0.9	4.2
Collection of fuel and wate	0.4	0.5	0.5

In addition to the enormous gender gaps observed for unpaid care work, for the total and the main components, the low participation and very limited time devoted by men and women to care of persons is worrying. It is less than 1 hour per day—slightly more than an hour for women and for men only 0.2 hours. While internationally childcare tends to be under-reported, including because it is often done simultaneously with other activities and is often perceived as a "responsibility" rather than "activity", considering the age structure of the Nicaraguan population and the almost non-existent supply of care services, whether public or market, this result suggests that younger people might be caring for themselves more than is desirable. This merits further in-depth study.

Figure 7.1 shows the distribution of time devoted to unpaid care work by the population in the 15–64 age group. As this figure indicates, nearly 50 per cent of men and 10 per cent of women devoted no time to this type of work during the reference day (the day prior to the interview). Between 1 and 120 minutes of unpaid care work is located 25 per cent of the men and 13.9 per cent of the women.

The concentration of men in the first groups, in terms of time devoted to unpaid care work, along with the fairly even distribution of women across the time groups (including the last ones), shows the profound gender inequality that exists in this area.

The distribution of time devoted to care for persons by the population in the 15–64 age group shows that 92.1 per cent and 63.5 per cent of men and women, respectively, stated that they had spent no time in care for persons (Figure 7.2). Thus, a majority of the population does not dedicate time to care for persons, whether children or individuals who are ill.

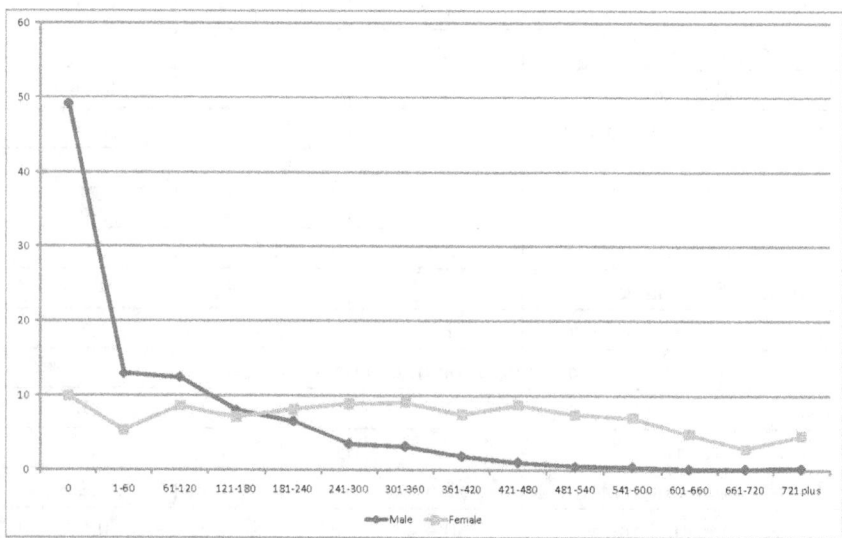

Figure 7.1 Distribution of time spent on unpaid care work by sex.

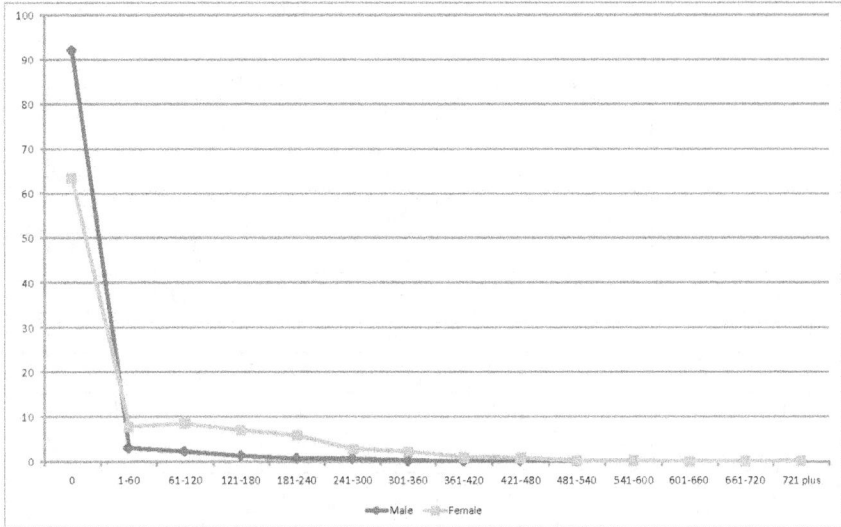

Figure 7.2 Distribution of time spent on care of persons by sex.

On the one hand, 7.9 per cent of the men who devoted time to care for persons were concentrated in the 1- to 120-minute group. On the other hand, 36.5 per cent of women who stated that they had cared for persons were in the 1- to 240-minute group.

Who Uses Time for What?

In this section we analyse the relationship between the use of time by men and women aged 15–64 years and selected socio-demographic and economic characteristics.

Men's rates of participation in SNA work and paid work are higher than women's in both urban and rural areas. Within the sexes, rural inhabitants show the highest participation rates in these types of work, suggesting that women have greater opportunities for paid work in the cities. The gender gap in these parameters is greater in the rural population.

Men also spend more hours per day in SNA work and paid work than do women. It is striking that it is in the rural population that the difference in time devoted to paid work (0.5 hours, or 6 per cent of the day) is the least pronounced.

The greatest difference between SNA work and paid work participation rates is seen among rural men, reflecting the extent to which they are active in the unpaid labour market.

As expected, women, and particularly rural women, show the largest amounts of time and highest rates of participation (over 90 per cent) in

Table 7.4 Participation Rates and Mean Time Spent by Population 15–64 Years on Selected Activities by Area of Residence and Sex

Area of residence and sex	Participation rate (%)			Mean time (hours per day)		
	SNA	Paid work	UCW	SNA	Paid work	UCW
Total	53.9	42.9	70.8	8.2	8.8	5.2
Male	74.9	60.2	50.8	8.5	9.0	3.0
Female	33.7	26.3	90.1	7.6	8.3	6.3
Urban	53.5	44.8	67.7	8.4	9.0	5.0
Male	67.7	57.9	44.4	8.8	9.3	2.9
Female	41.4	33.8	87.3	7.8	8.4	5.8
Rural	54.5	40.7	74.5	8.1	8.5	5.4
Male	82.2	62.4	57.2	8.3	8.6	3.0
Female	23.3	16.3	93.8	7.1	8.1	7.0

unpaid care work. Independent of area of residence, they devote twice as long to these activities than do men. Among men, it is rural inhabitants who are most involved in unpaid care work, a phenomenon that may reflect the inclusion of water collection and firewood gathering, though the time they spend is comparable to that spent by their urban counterparts.

Rural women devote 20 per cent more time than urban women to unpaid care work, probably due to their poorer housing conditions and the greater number of members per household. However, the data suggest that these factors do not affect men's behaviour.

Rates of participation in SNA work and paid work show marked differences from one age group to another. Both sexes show the highest participation rates in the 31–49 year group, followed by the 50–64 year group, the 18–30 year and the 15–17 year age groups. The average time devoted by men and women shows a similar pattern.

As shown in Table 7.5, the greatest gender difference in SNA work is seen in the 18–30 year age group, followed very closely by the 50–64 year group, which also exhibits the greatest difference between men's and women's participation in paid work. In terms of time devoted by the two sexes to these types of work, however, the greatest difference is seen in the 15–17 year group.

The difference between rates of participation in SNA work and paid work diminishes with advancing age in both men and women, which could indicate that the proportion of unpaid market work diminishes with age.

Women's participation rates in unpaid care work do not vary significantly by age group, although slightly higher values are found in the 18–30 and 31–49 year groups, which are precisely the groups in which men's participation rates are lowest. The time that men devote to unpaid care work

Table 7.5 Participation Rates and Mean Time Spent by Population 15–64 Years on Selected Activities by Age Group and Sex

Age group and sex	Participation rate (%)			Mean time (hours per day)		
	SNA	Paid work	UCW	SNA	Paid work	UCW
Total	53.9	42.9	70.8	8.2	8.8	5.2
15–17 years	33.8	17.0	71.8	7.2	8.2	4.5
Male	50.2	25.5	54.8	7.8	8.5	3.0
Female	17.0	8.3	89.3	5.6	7.3	5.5
18–30 years	53.5	40.2	70.3	8.2	8.8	5.3
Male	75.7	57.3	49.5	8.5	9.0	2.9
Female	31.6	23.4	90.7	7.4	8.4	6.6
31–49 years	62.7	55.5	71.3	8.5	8.9	5.3
Male	84.8	76.4	49.5	8.8	9.1	3.0
Female	43.1	36.9	90.5	8.0	8.4	6.4
50–64 years	56.3	49.3	70.3	8.3	8.7	4.9
Male	77.9	70.4	53.1	8.6	8.8	2.9
Female	34.0	27.6	88.0	7.7	8.2	6.2

is practically invariant with age (2.9 hours per day), and although women's time varies little, it is twice that spent by men.

As Table 7.6 shows, participation in SNA work and paid work is greatest among men who are married or in conjugal unions and separated/divorced/widowed women, while the lowest rates are among single men and women.

As concerns time devoted to SNA work, men who are married or in conjugal unions, along with separated/divorced/widowed women, report the highest figures, while the lowest are among single persons of both sexes. For paid work, the highest times are reported by men who are married or in conjugal unions and separated/divorced/widowed men, and by women who are married or in conjugal unions and single women. The lowest times are reported by single men and separated/divorced/widowed women.

In unpaid care work, women's participation rates are higher than men's by at least 50 per cent, and the differential is nearly 100 per cent among the population that is married or in conjugal unions. Separated/divorced/widowed men are most involved in unpaid care work—most likely driven by the lack of a partner—while those who are married or in conjugal unions and single men are least involved. Women who are married or in conjugal unions show the highest rates of participation in unpaid care work, and single women show the lowest. This confirms that the likelihood of doing unpaid care work increases with being female, with having a family, with

Table 7.6 Participation Rates and Mean Time Spent by Population 15–64 Years on Selected Activities by Conjugal Status and Sex

Conjugal status	Participation rate (%)			Mean time (hours per day)		
	SNA	Paid work	UCW	SNA	Paid work	UCW
Total	53.9	42.9	70.8	8.2	8.8	5.2
Married or in conjugal union	58.2	51.0	71.8	8.5	8.9	5.6
Male	84.7	77.1	50.0	8.8	9.0	3.0
Female	32.2	25.4	93.2	7.7	8.4	7.0
Separated, divorced, widowed	52.8	44.0	82.5	8.0	8.5	5.6
Male	75.4	60.0	59.0	8.5	8.9	3.4
Female	46.0	39.2	89.6	7.8	8.2	6.0
Single	46.0	27.5	63.2	7.8	8.6	3.9
Male	60.3	34.8	50.5	8.0	8.7	2.9
Female	25.2	16.0	83.2	7.0	8.4	4.9

having a conjugal partner in the case of women, and with not having a stable partner in the case of men.

The greatest time devoted to unpaid care work is seen among separated/divorced/widowed men, and among women in conjugal unions, with the lowest rate being among single men and women as well as men in conjugal unions. These data suggest that for women who have their own family, having a conjugal partner increases unpaid work time, while this situation decreases unpaid work time for men.

As Table 7.7 shows, men's participation in SNA work and paid work increases with the presence of children under age 6 in the household, especially when there are two or more children, while women's participation in SNA work decreases. There is a slight tendency for the amount of time that men devote to these types of work to increase with an increase in the number of children in the household. For women, the average time devoted to SNA work and paid work increases from the no-children to one-child group (6 per cent and 3 per cent, respectively, for the two types of work), but diminishes by 10 per cent when there are 2 or more children in the household.

In regard to unpaid care work, men's and women's participation rates diminish when the number of children in the household increases from 0 to 1, then increases again when there are 2 or more. The time that men devote to care work follows a pattern similar to that described previously for participation rates. In contrast, women's time clearly increases.

It would seem, then, that the presence of children under 6 in the household leads to a reinforcement or resumption of traditional gender roles,

Nicaragua 185

Table 7.7 Participation Rates and Mean Time Spent by Population 15–64 Years on Selected Activities by Sex and Number of Children Under 6 Years in Household

Sex and number of children under 6 years	Participation rate (%)			Mean time (hours per day)		
	SNA	Paid work	UCW	SNA	Paid work	UCW
Total	53.9	42.9	70.8	8.2	8.8	5.2
Male	74.9	60.1	50.8	8.5	9.0	3.0
None	69.5	56.3	55.3	8.4	8.9	3.2
One child	71.5	57.5	47.8	8.4	9.0	2.8
Two or more	76.4	61.2	50.7	8.6	9.0	3.0
Female	33.7	26.3	90.1	7.6	8.3	6.3
None	42.4	32.9	89.0	7.8	8.7	5.2
One child	33.2	28.1	86.0	8.3	9.0	5.9
Two or more	33.0	25.4	91.0	7.4	8.2	6.5

as women reduce their participation in paid work to devote more time to unpaid care work, whereas men do the opposite.

As might be expected, the employed population of both sexes reports the highest participation rates and average time devoted to SNA work and paid work. For both types of work, the greatest differences between men's and women's rates are among the unemployed. However, it would be inadvisable to draw any conclusion from this, since this segment represents less than 7 per cent f the total population in the 15–64 age group, and shows participation rates below 5 per cent.

Unemployed men and economically inactive women are the most involved in unpaid care work—69.0 per cent and 95.5 per cent, respectively. However, unemployed and employed women's participation rates are high (92.4 per cent and 82.2 per cent), which indicates that these women are doing both types of work. Employed men and women show the lowest participation rates (48.2 per cent and 82.2 per cent). Unemployed men and economically inactive women devote the most time to unpaid care work (4.1 and 7.3 hours per day, respectively). Employed men and women show the lowest amounts of time (2.8 hours and 4.7 hours per day, respectively).

Men's and women's participation in SNA work and paid work diminishes as household income increases, although the pattern is clearer for women (Table 7.9). The very limited participation of first-quintile women in paid work is striking.

As regards time spent in SNA work, there is a tendency for men to do less as one moves from quintile 1 to quintile 5. The pattern for women fluctuates, both increasing and diminishing as one moves from one quintile to

186 Isolda Espinosa González

Table 7.8 Participation Rates and Mean Time Spent by Population 15–64 Years on Selected Activities by Activity Status and Sex

Activity status	Participation rate (%)			Mean time (hours per day)		
	SNA	Paid work	UCW	SNA	Paid work	UCW
Total	53.9	42.9	70.8	8.2	8.8	5.2
Employed	83.9	70.4	59.5	8.5	8.8	3.7
Male	87.1	72.7	48.2	8.7	9.0	2.8
Female	77.4	65.9	82.2	8.0	8.4	4.7
Unemployed	28.2	4.7	79.3	5.2	7.9	5.3
Male	36.1	5.6	69.0	5.7	8.1	4.1
Female	18.2	3.5	92.4	4.0	7.6	6.4
Inactive	4.1	0.0	89.8	3.6	0.0	6.9
Male	6.1	0.0	57.8	3.9	0.0	3.2
Female	3.7	0.0	95.5	3.5	0.0	7.3

the next. The time spent by both sexes in paid work increases along with household income.

In terms of unpaid care work, there is a clear pattern of diminishing participation rates among both men and women with increasing household income. A similar pattern is seen in the time devoted by both sexes to this type of work, although the pattern is more pronounced among women. As mentioned before, these patterns, particularly evident among women, suggest that domestic workers in the household are assuming some of the care burden.

WHAT ARE THE PARTICIPATION RATES FOR CARE?

Just as one commonly estimates the "rate of economic dependency", the UNRISD project on the Political and Social Economy of Care developed the rate of care dependency. As discussed in Chapter 1, this is defined as the proportion of the population that, on account of its age (under 15 years and more than 64 years) is likely to depend on care provided by people aged 15–64 years, who are considered capable of caring both for themselves and, in addition, caring for younger and older people.

Table 7.10 reveals that the care dependency rate for Nicaragua is 0.61. That is, each person providing care is responsible for more than half of the care needed by a dependant person. The age group 0–6 years contributes the most to the care dependency rate, followed by the group aged 7–12 years. This is consistent with the demographic trend of the last decades in which fertility has fallen, but the level remains relatively high.

Nicaragua records the highest care dependency rate when compared with the other countries covered by the UNRISD project.

Table 7.9 Participation Rates and Mean Time Spent by Population 15–64 Years on Selected Activities by Sex and Monetary Household Income Quintile

Monetary household income quintile and sex	Participation rate (%)			Mean time (hours per day)		
	SNA	Paid work	UCW	SNA	Paid work	UCW
Total	53.9	42.9	70.8	8.1	8.2	5.2
Quintile 1	49.3	30.5	81.4	8.4	7.7	5.6
Male	84.4	55.3	67.2	8.9	8.0	3.1
Female	16.2	7.2	94.8	8.0	6.0	7.4
Quintile 2	51.8	40.0	75.5	8.5	8.1	5.6
Male	76.8	59.5	56.9	8.4	8.4	3.4
Female	27.8	21.2	93.8	8.6	7.5	6.9
Quintile 3	52.6	44.0	72.7	7.9	8.3	5.0
Male	72.8	61.1	52.2	7.8	8.7	2.8
Female	32.6	26.9	93.0	8.1	7.3	6.2
Quintile 4	54.8	46.8	67.8	8.0	8.3	5.1
Male	71.0	60.7	45.5	7.4	8.6	2.8
Female	39.4	33.8	89.0	8.5	7.6	6.1
Quintile 5	58.6	48.3	62.2	7.8	8.5	4.6
Male	73.0	62.3	40.0	7.5	8.8	2.7
Female	44.6	34.9	83.6	8.2	8.1	5.5

Table 7.10 Care Dependency Ratio

	Age group	Population 1995	Weight	Weighted population	%
A	1–6	970,547	1.0	970,547.0	26.7
B	7–12	753,197	0.5	376,598.5	10.3
C	75–84	45,269	0.5	22,634.5	0.6
D	85 plus	16,247	1.0	16,247.0	0.5
E	15–74	2,254,956	1.0	2,254,956.0	61.9
	Total	4,040,216		3,640,983.0	100.0

Care dependency ratio = (A+B+C+D)/E = 0.61

MULTIVARIATE ANALYSIS OF TIME USE

How do the preceding variables combine to influence the number of hours spent on unpaid care work in general and care of persons in particular?

To answer this question we use the Tobit model of censured regression, as discussed in Chapter 1. In the following section we present two Tobit estimates, the first for unpaid care work and the second for care of persons. The definition of unpaid care work used includes the care of persons, domestic chores and collection of fuel and water.

We define unpaid care work as the dependent variable, and explore the factors that can explain it. The explanatory factors considered are sex (being male), age, age squared, being a child (6–17 years), place of residence (rural area), marital status (being partnered or married), the presence of someone less than 6 years of age in the household, household income and the natural logarithm of household income.

Unpaid Care Work

All of the variables except being a child and household income are found to be significant at the 95 per cent confidence interval, but the natural logarithm of household income is significant.

Being male has the strongest effect (highest coefficient in absolute terms) on the amount of unpaid care work done. The amount of unpaid care work tends to decrease if the person is male, and as log household income increases. The coefficient of age is positive while that of age-squared is negative. This implies that the time spent on unpaid care work initially increases with age but afterwards declines. All the remaining variables tend to result in an increase in the amount of unpaid care work done. The corrected r^2 of 29 per cent implies that the explanatory power of the model is relatively low.

Based on the aforementioned, we can say that in Nicaragua those who spend most time on unpaid care work are women, rural residents, those who are married or partners, members of households where the natural logarithm of household income is lower, and households which include a child under 6 years of age. The amount of unpaid care work initially increases with age, but then declines.

Care of Persons

In this case the time dedicated to care of persons is defined as the dependent variable while the independent variables from the previous model are maintained.

Table 7.12 suggests that age and household income are not significant at the 5 per cent level of confidence. Of the significant variables, being male, being a child (6–17 years), being in a conjugal relationship and the number of members less than 6 years of age in the household have the most influence over the time spent on childcare. The first two reduce the amount of time while the last two increase it.

Table 7.11 Tobit Estimation of Unpaid Care Work

Variable	Coefficient	Standard error	t	P>|t|	95% confidence interval	
Male	-4.3127380	0.0945324	-45.62	0.000	-4.4980460	-4.1274300
Rural	0.69731112	0.1009744	6.91	0.000	0.4993756	0.8952467
Married/in conjugal union	0.5814599	0.1224893	4.75	0.000	0.3413496	0.8215703
ln household income	-0.5603796	0.0575888	-9.73	0.000	-0.6732683	-0.4474908
Children under age 6 in household	0.2602167	0.0402794	6.46	0.000	0.1812588	0.3391746
Age	0.1921783	0.0157332	12.21	0.000	0.1613372	0.2230193
Age squared	-0.0022111	0.0001724	-12.82	0.000	-0.0025491	-0.0018731
Child	0.0877233	0.1884553	0.47	0.642	-0.2816973	0.4571439
Household income	0.0000053	0.0000169	0.31	0.754	-0.0000278	0.0000384
Constant	4.4116400	0.5120024	8.62	0.000	3.4079850	5.4152960
Sigma	3.9348890	0.0301251			3.8562330	4.0135440

Table 7.12 Tobit Estimation of Care of Persons

Variable	Coefficient	Standard error	t	P > |t|	95% confidence interval	
Male	-3.8706670	0.1658004	-23.35	0.000	-4.1956780	-3.5456560
Child	-1.6696470	0.2897171	-5.76	0.000	-2.2375660	-1.1017270
Married/in conjugal union	1.1743890	0.1762326	6.66	0.000	0.8289277	1.5198500
Children under age 6 in household	0.8464503	0.0583250	14.51	0.000	0.7321183	0.9607823
Rural	-0.5256437	0.1529992	-3.44	0.001	-0.8255612	-0.2257263
Age squared	-0.0009105	0.0002812	-3.24	0.001	-0.0014617	-0.0003592
ln household income	-0.1652479	0.0888587	-1.86	0.063	-0.3394337	0.0089380
Age	0.0445207	0.0247253	1.80	0.072	-0.0039472	0.0929886
Household income	-0.0000043	0.0000278	-0.15	0.878	-0.0000588	0.0000503
Constant	-2.0983930	0.7885966	-2.66	0.008	-3.6442440	-0.5525419
Sigma	4.1942610	0.0917088			4.0144880	4.3740330

Taken as a whole, this model explains 33.3 per cent (r^2 corrected = 0.3316378) of the variation in the dependent variable, which, although a higher coefficient than the previous model, still represents a very low explanatory capacity. Nevertheless, we must bear in mind that a small value for r^2 does not necessarily imply that it is not a good model.

In summary, in Nicaragua, the people who invest most time in care of persons are women, older than 17 years, married or partners, members of households which include a member less than six years, and those residing in rural areas.

WHAT IS THE VALUE OF UNPAID CARE WORK IN NICARAGUA?

This section provides an estimate of the value of unpaid care work and some of its components, in order to arrive at an approximation of this hidden cost of production, which is not recognised in the SNA, and to make visible women's contribution to the national economy. The procedure described in Chapter 1 is followed. The estimation methods used were median income and the generalist or replacement cost approach.

The median income method (as its name suggests) uses the median income for the entire population. For purposes of the present document, median income was calculated on the basis of the data in the economic activity section of the 1998 EMNV. The income of the employed population was considered, regardless of whether this involved wage workers, own-account workers or business owners. Only unpaid workers and those not reporting labour income were excluded. Recognising income differences by sex, the figures were calculated separately for men and women.

Though we realise that respondents tend to seriously understate their income, we did not adjust the 1998 EMNV data to reflect this. This decision was based on the difficulties involved in determining the magnitude of the overall adjustment required, as well as the impossibility of identifying individual incomes that were understated in a survey of this type.

The generalist or replacement cost method is based on the cost of replacing unpaid care work by the paid services of a person responsible for performing all such work. The services of this person are assumed to be remunerated at the median wage for the occupation involved. The occupation chosen for this purpose was domestic work; thus, the figure used was the median wage for domestic employees.

In determining remuneration of domestic employees, both monetary and estimated in-kind payments were considered, since the latter component represents a significant element in this occupation. In this case, we also used the median and the adjusted average[7] of the reported remuneration.

As Table 7.13 shows, in this case the value of unpaid care work is between C$11,606.76 million and C$20,531.37 million, depending on the approach and statistics used. The estimated value for unpaid care for persons is between C$2,060.61 million and C$3,629.39 million. Women account for approximately 79 per cent of the value of unpaid care work and 87 per cent of the value of care of persons.

In order to assess the meaning of the different estimates of unpaid care work and unpaid care for persons, we now examine these in relation to some key economic variables.

As Table 7.14 indicates, the value of unpaid care work is equivalent to 30.7 per cent of gross domestic product (GDP) if the median wage of domestic employees is used as a measure of value, and 54.3 per cent if the average income of employed men and women is used. The estimated value of unpaid care for persons represents between 5.5 per cent and 9.6 per cent of GDP, according to the approach and statistic selected. The estimated value of care of persons done by women aged 15–64 years is equivalent to 4.7 per cent and 8.3 per cent of GDP.

Table 7.13 Estimated Value of Unpaid Care Work and Care of Persons for the Population 15–64 years, 1998 (Millions Córdobas)

	UCW			Care of persons		
	Total	Male	Female	Total	Male	Female
Average income of employed by sex approach						
Total value (adjusted average)	20,531.37	4,417.16	16,114.21	3,629.39	493.22	3,136.18
Generalist approach (domestic employee wage)						
Total value (median)	11,606.76	2,390.46	9,216.30	2,060.61	266.92	1,793.69
Total value (adjusted average)	13,192.78	2,717.11	10,475.67	2,342.18	303.39	2,038.79

Table 7.14 Value of Unpaid Care Work and Care of Persons of the Population 15–64 Years Compared to Gross Domestic Product, 1998 (per cent)

	UCW			Care of persons		
	Total	Male	Female	Total	Male	Female
Average income approach	54.3	11.7	42.6	9.6	1.3	8.3
Generalist approach						
Median	30.7	6.3	24.4	5.4	0.7	4.7
Average	34.9	7.2	27.7	6.2	0.8	5.4

Using data from other sections of the 1998 EMNV, we can also compare the value of unpaid care work and care of persons with the value of paid work in the economy. For this purpose, we have considered only monetary income received by men and women as wage-earners, as own-account workers and as business owners. Unpaid workers are not included.

We find that the value of unpaid care work is either almost the same as (107.4 per cent of) or approximately double (190.0 per cent of) the value of paid work, according to which estimating method is used. Meanwhile, the value of unpaid care for persons represents between 19.1 per cent and 33.6 per cent of the value of paid work. Comparing these two types of work by sex, however, reveals major differences.

For men, the value of unpaid care work represents between 22.1 per cent and 56.5 per cent of the value of paid work. Among women, on the other hand, the figure is between 85.3 per cent and 539.6 per cent. The value of unpaid care for persons provided by men represents only between 2.5 per cent and 6.3 per cent of the value of paid work, while the value of this type of work done by women is between 16.6 per cent and 105.0 per cent.

Comparing with tax, the value of unpaid care work in 1998 represented between approximately two and four times the value of total tax revenue. When the comparison is with income tax revenue, the factor is very much greater: between 1,562.7 per cent and 2,764.2 per cent, due primarily to the relatively low importance of income tax (and direct taxes in general) in the Nicaraguan tax system. The value of unpaid care for persons represents between 38.9 per cent and 68.6 per cent of total tax revenue, and between 277.4 per cent and 488.6 per cent of income tax revenue.

Finally, we calculate the value of unpaid care work and unpaid care for persons as a percentage of the amount budgeted by the central government in 1998 for salaries in the Ministry of Education, Ministry of Health and Ministry of Social Affairs. In 1988, the national territory was demarcated into regions, departments and municipalities, all of which were subordinate to the executive branch both administratively and financially. The Municipal Law of 2 July 1988 established the competencies of these entities, which did not include education, health or social security. The central ministry budgets thus provide a good approximation of government spending on social services.

Taking the smallest estimate of the value of unpaid care work (the median under the generalist approach), we find that it represents 4,353.1 per cent, 2,894.5 per cent and 360,890.5 per cent of salaries for the Ministries of Education, Health and Social Affairs, respectively. If the same calculation is done for unpaid care for persons, the resulting figures are 772.8 per cent, 513.9 per cent and 64,070.7 per cent. These enormous magnitudes largely reflect the central government's low level of social spending (one of the lowest in Latin America), particularly in the areas studied; and confirm the assessment of the political social regime in Nicaragua as residual and its welfare regime as highly familialist.

CONCLUSION

The data analysed clearly point to a set of patterns—a number of which were to be expected—in the ways Nicaraguans aged 15 to 64 years old distribute their time between paid work and unpaid care work. Among these we highlight the following:

- On the one hand, more men than women participate in paid work and they dedicate more time to it
- More women, on the other hand, engage in unpaid childcare, and they devote more hours per day to it than do men
- Area of residence barely influences the participation of men in paid work, but does so for women. Urban women residents engage more and devote more time to paid work than rural women
- Urban men's participation in unpaid care work is slightly higher than the rate for rural men, though the number of hours per day is the same for the two groups
- More men and women in the 18–49 age group engage in paid work, and they devote more time to it
- Men engage in unpaid care work more in the declining phase of their work lives. In contrast, women do so more at the peak of their labour capacity, suggesting competing pressures in terms of time use
- Being in conjugal unions increases the probability of women's being involved in unpaid care work, and decreases their likelihood of doing paid work. For men, the pattern is the reverse
- The presence of children under age 6 in the household seems to impel men toward paid work, and to prevent women from performing it. Nevertheless, the presence of these younger children in the household does not affect the time that men spend on unpaid care work, but instead that invested by women
- Being employed does not free women from their responsibility for unpaid care work. Although they devote less time to this work than other women, the number of hours per day they spend (approximately 4) is hardly negligible, indicating that employed women face a work overload
- Household income levels are positively correlated with men's and women's rates of participation in paid work. The opposite is true in regard to women in unpaid care work. That is, at high levels of household income the involvement of men and women in paid work is greater, with less involvement in unpaid care work, which could be associated with the presence of domestic workers in the household and/or the use of nursery or pre-school services for the care of the children

The multiple regression analysis confirmed that the amount of time spent on unpaid care work and care of persons depends on sex, area of residence, marital status and the presence of children under 6 years of age in the household. Sex is the most influential factor in both cases.

The preceding suggests the persistence of traditional conceptions of gender that assign to men the role of household provider and to women that of caregiver, despite the fact that a significant proportion of women—including those with partners and children—are involved in paid work and play the role of providers for the household, given the need to have an additional income to satisfy household needs. However, men—especially those between 18 and 49 years—do not participate equivalently in unpaid care work, resulting in employed women being overburdened with work.

One surprising finding was the small time spent by men and women on care of person. Given the age structure of the Nicaraguan population and the almost non-existent supply of care services, whether public or market, this suggests that a large proportion of younger people care for themselves. To the ethical problems, of respect for and promotion of the rights of the child that this situation raises, are added the new capacities demanded of the labour force. This does not simply concern training in the use of new technologies, but also new personal and emotional skills to enable rapid adaptation to the changes caused by globalisation. In other words, generational reproduction requires more care work than before to avoid exclusion.

The most conservative estimate of the value of unpaid care work is equivalent to 30.7 per cent of GDP, 80 per cent of which is accounted for by women. However, the capacity of women to absorb the costs of economic policies or the growth in demand for care is not infinite. If we want to formulate public policies that have sustainable human development as their objective, we cannot ignore this reality. The need thus arises to continue generating information and analysis of the use of time of Nicaraguans, which can influence decision-making and improvement of the relationship between the state and Nicaraguan society.

NOTES

1. The term "social reproduction" is used to refer broadly to the reproduction of the ideological and material conditions that sustain a social system. "Reproduction of the work force" refers to the daily maintenance of workers and future workers, as well as to the process of educating and training them. "Unpaid care work" is a similar concept.
2. Although the time use section of the 1998 EMNV included questions referring specifically to these categories, it also included two questions on family economic activity (both agricultural and non-agricultural), but without inquiring as to whether remuneration was received. To deal at least partially with this situation, we consulted the economic activity section of the survey and used its classification scheme to categorise activities as paid or unpaid.
3. Nicaragua's legislation grants equal rights to all couples, regardless of the type of conjugal union of which they are a part.

4. According to the Encuesta de Demografía y Salud [Demographic and Health Survey] (ENDESA), the median age of any first unions was 18.2 years in 2001.
5. The poverty line is defined in terms of the monthly per capita consumption needed to satisfy minimum caloric requirements (the extreme poverty line), plus an additional amount to cover consumption of essential non-food goods and services, such as housing, transportation, education, health and clothing, as well as daily household expenses.
6. According to official 1998 data, 47.9 per cent of the country's population was under the consumption poverty line.
7. The adjusted average is calculated without including the extreme values (2.5 per cent at each extreme).

REFERENCES

Carrasco, Cristina. 2006. "La Economía Feminista: Una Apuesta por Otra Economía" (mimeo).

Picchio, Antonella. 1999. "Visibilidad Analítica y Política del Trabajo de Reproducción Social." In Cristina Carrasco (ed.), *Mujeres y Economía*. Icaria, Madrid.

Picchio, Antonella. 1994. "El Trabajo de Reproducción, Tema Central en el Análisis del Mercado Laboral." In C. Borderías, C. Carrasco, C. Alemany (ed.), *Las Mujeres y el Trabajo. Rupturas Conceptuales*. Icaria, Madrid.

Rodríguez Enríquez, Corina. 2005. *Economía del Cuidado y Política Económica: Una Aproximación a sus Interrelaciones* (Draft). Economic Commission for Latin America and the Caribbean. Document for the 38th meeting of the Presiding Officers of the Regional Conference on Women in Latin America and the Caribbean. Mar del Plata, Argentina, 7–8 September, 2005.

8 Unpaid Care Work in the City of Buenos Aires

Valeria Esquivel

THE BUENOS AIRES TIME USE SURVEY AS A TOOL TO ANALYSE UNPAID CARE WORK

The Buenos Aires Time Use Survey was conducted by the Directorate-General of Statistics of the City Government (Dirección General de Estadística y Censos, DGEyC) as a module of the City of Buenos Aires' Annual Household Survey in November-December 2005.[1] Information for the survey was collected under a cooperation agreement between DGEyC and Instituto de Ciencias, Universidad Nacional de General Sarmiento, Argentina.

The survey's primary purpose was to quantify unpaid care work, performed by (mostly) women and (some) men for their households and communities, on an unremunerated basis. Survey results show gender inequalities in the distribution of unpaid care work, which combine with other dimensions of inequality—such as class, generation and family structure—to impact on women's and households' opportunities and material well-being. Ultimately, the Buenos Aires Time Use Survey aimed at providing the women's movement and politicians alike with a powerful tool to advocate for, and promote, policies that enhance the situation of women and contribute to the equitable integration of women and men into society.

The Buenos Aires Time Use Survey was the first to be collected in the country following the publication of United Nations guidelines (UNSD 2005). It is also a unique experience in the Latin American context since, despite being a module attached to an ongoing multi-purpose household survey, it departed from the widely used short tasks list approach to collecting time use data by using the 24-hour recall activity diary (Esquivel 2008). Its design drew heavily on the activity diary applied in the 2000 South African time use survey, although a closer look reveals a number of methodological variations, particularly with respect to the activity classification and the way simultaneous activities were captured (Budlender 2007).

Although there is no space here to provide a detailed review of the survey's methodology (which can be found in Esquivel, 2010), it should be stressed that the 24-hour recall activity diary proved to be particularly well-suited for capturing unpaid care work. By allowing for up to three non-hierarchical simultaneous activities, the 24-hour recall diary provided for capturing unpaid care work which is performed in parallel with other activities and which might otherwise be omitted from reporting when socially more valued activities take place at the same time. Also, asking pair-wise whether each activity was performed (or not) simultaneously with other/s made it possible to assign more exact "full-minute" times to each activity, i.e. the total time spent on the activity irrespective of its being performed simultaneously with others. Alternatively, "24-hour" times could also be calculated, for which the sum of the times devoted to all activities in a day is exactly 24 hours. Fully considering simultaneity "extended" the average day by 4:30 hours for women and 4 hours for men, proving that simultaneity is an essential feature of time use in Argentina (DGEyC 2007b).

ANALYSING UNPAID CARE WORKING TIME IN THE CITY OF BUENOS AIRES

In this chapter, activities categorised under household maintenance (coded under 400), care of persons (500), and unpaid community work (600) in the Buenos Aires Classification of Time Use Activities are all considered part of unpaid care work (DGEyC 2005a).

SNA work theoretically includes unpaid production of goods for own consumption, and fetching wood and collecting water. However, none of these activities were differentiated in the Buenos Aires Classification of Time Use Activities, given the fact that the City of Buenos Aires is a massive urban centre.

The Buenos Aires Time Use Survey is representative of the City of Buenos Aires 15- to 74- year-old population living in households,[2] namely 2.135 million people; 55 per cent of them female and 45 per cent male.

Aside from the time use information, the Buenos Aires Time Use Survey includes demographic and socioeconomic information both for the individual and for her/his household. Among the many standard individual characteristics that can be identified, this chapter presents tables by sex; age (which is collected in years); educational attainment; labour market status (inactive, unemployed, or employed); and relationship to household head (head, spouse, daughter/son, other members).

In Argentina's statistical system, the head of household is determined by whoever the respondent names as the "head", or whoever is designated by family members as such (rather than some objective criteria, such as who is the main income earner). In practice most heads of households would also be the ones earning the higher incomes.[3] Nearly 70 per cent of men are heads of household, and only a small percentage report being spouse or partner. In contrast, 50 per cent of women report that they are spouse or partner, and only 32 per cent report being head of household. Of the latter (i.e. women who are heads), one third are heads of one-person households.

Household characteristics analysed in this chapter are household type; presence and age of children; and household absolute poverty. The household types used are relatively sophisticated and have been built based on kinship relationships to capture more fully the functioning of families. Non-family households are one-person households and non-family multi-person households.

Household types

One-person household: Head of household only.[4]
Couple without children: Head of household and spouse.
Complete nuclear family with daughters/sons: Couple with at least one unmarried daughter/son (most of them are children, but could be 18 years or older).
Partial nuclear family (one-parent): Single parent with at least one unmarried daughter/son.
Extended family: Head of household or nuclear family plus other relative/s of head of household;
Other: Complex households (head of household, nuclear family or extended family, plus non-family member(s)) and non-family multi-person households (head of household and non-family member(s).

The structure of the weighted sample by household type shows the predominance of nuclear-family households: six out of ten inhabitants of the city who are between the ages of 15 and 74 live in nuclear-family households (couples without children and complete nuclear families with children). The percentage is smaller among women (56 per cent) than among men (64 per cent). Also, over four out of ten Buenos Aires residents between 15 and 74 years of age live in households with at least one child (under 18), while 17 per cent of the city's total population lives in households with at least one child aged 5 years or younger.

Household income information is of inferior quality compared to the information presented in the preceding paragraph—it represents only 1.748 million people, due to a (relatively high) non-response rate to family income (18 per cent). Household income information allows calculation of the absolute poverty rate, with poverty defined as the lack of sufficient income to purchase what is considered a basic bundle of goods. The population living below the poverty line in the City of Buenos Aires at the time the Buenos Aires Time Use Survey was conducted (second half of 2005) stood at 11.5 per cent, which is substantially lower than the rate for the country as a whole (33.8 per cent) in the same period. Non-response rates and the limitations of sampling design that did not reach the city's most vulnerable groups (living in boarding houses and shanty towns) explain

200 *Valeria Esquivel*

why the Buenos Aires Time Use Survey poverty rate is even lower, at only 7 per cent.

SNA WORK, UNPAID CARE WORK AND CARE OF PERSONS

On average, the proportion of total time devoted to productive activities (SNA work plus unpaid care work) does not differ much between women and men aged 15–74 years living in the city of Buenos Aires: productive activities take up 7:02 hours (24-hours) for women and 6:48 hours for men. However, gender-based differences emerge powerfully in productive activities as women and men distribute their work burdens in highly dissimilar ways.

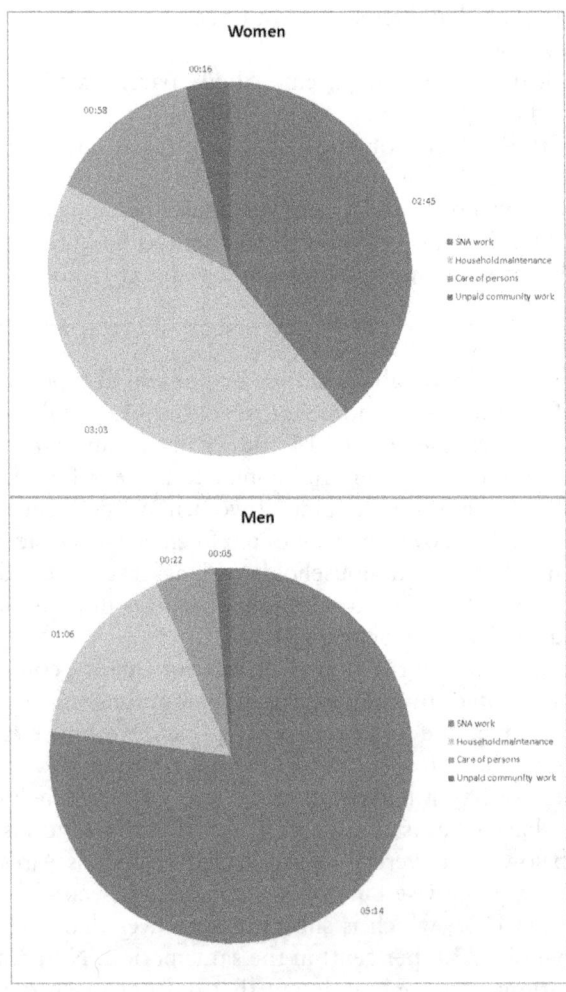

Figure 8.1 Composition of total working time (24-hours) by sex.

Figure 8.1 shows that over three-fourths of men's mean working time is devoted to SNA work, while only one third of women's mean working time is devoted to the same (primarily) market-oriented activities. The mean time used by women for household maintenance, care of persons and unpaid services to the community is triple that used by men.

In what follows, mean time spent in SNA work and unpaid care work is compared for different population groups. Tables also show care of persons in detail, to highlight its relative size within unpaid care work. All times are expressed in hours and minutes, and refer to mean population times (24 hour time). Totals correspond to those in Figure 8.1 and are repeated in all tables. When the size of a particular population group is too small to allow for a (statistically) significant estimation of time, this is indicated in a note to the relevant table.[5]

In the tables that follow, adding times in horizontal cells pair-wise for the SNA work and the unpaid care work columns gives an idea of the mean total working time that women, men or the total population perform in a given day. For example, adding 2:45 hours of women's SNA work to 4:18 of unpaid care work results in the aforementioned 7:02 hours of productive work by women, while adding 5:14 hours of men's SNA work to their 1:33 hours of unpaid care work results in men's mean working time (6:48) (figures taken from the Total row in Table 8.1 and successive tables). This horizontal sum should not include the last group of columns, as care of persons is a sub-set of the unpaid care work.

Starting with the analysis by age group, it is clear that the young work the least (SNA work plus unpaid care work) on average, while those above retirement age (65 to 74 years old), as expected, perform less SNA work.

Table 8.1 Mean Time Spent in SNA Work, Unpaid Care Work and Care of Persons, by Sex and Age

	SNA work			Unpaid care work			Care of persons		
	Total	Women	Men	Total	Women	Men	Total	Women	Men
Total	03:52	02:45	05:14	03:04	04:18	01:33	00:41	00:58	00:22
Age 15 to 24	01:43	01:20	02:01	01:08	01:50	00:36	00:12	00:21	00:05
Age 25 to 39	05:08	03:58	06:36	03:34	04:46	02:03	01:30	02:03	00:49
Age 40 to 49	04:58	02:50	07:34	03:23	04:44	01:46	00:55	01:10	00:36
Age 50 to 64	04:13	03:02	06:05	03:27	04:43	01:25	00:18	00:27	00:04
Age 65 to 74	01:35	00:50	02:39	03:37	04:33	02:19	00:06	00:11	00:01

Women and men in the middle age bracket (25 to 39 years old) are the ones who work most; adding SNA work to unpaid care work results in total working times of 8:45 and 8:39 for women and men respectively. Relatively high mean times for unpaid care work for women and men in this age bracket are related to the highest times devoted to care of persons, of over two hours in the case of women and 0:49 minutes in the case of men.

Patterns of SNA work do not change that much for prime-age men, as mean times peak between the ages of 40 and 49 and only decrease after retirement age (65 years old). Women use the equivalent of roughly two-thirds of men's time on SNA work between the ages of 15 to 24 and between the ages of 25 to 39, when women's mean SNA working time peaks.

With the exception of young women, all other women devote a substantial number of hours (just under 5 hours) to unpaid care work. Interestingly, these consistently high times are accompanied by varying times for care of persons, which suggests that forms of unpaid care work other than care of persons—household maintenance and/or unpaid community work—must be varying with age.

Men reach a peak in their unpaid care work time after retirement age, while their time spent on care of persons reaches a peak between 25 and 39 years of age. Women and men above retirement age perform very little——if any—care of persons, possibly because many of them become care recipients.

Table 8.2 Mean Time Spent in SNA Work, Unpaid Care Work and Care of Persons, by Sex and Educational Level

	SNA work			Unpaid care work			Care of persons		
	Total	Women	Men	Total	Women	Men	Total	Women	Men
Total	03:52	02:45	05:14	03:04	04:18	01:33	00:41	00:58	00:22
Secondary not completed	03:25	02:10	04:53	03:11	04:30	01:40	00:33	00:46	00:18
Completed secondary/ university not completed	03:19	02:23	04:24	02:51	04:01	01:32	00:39	00:51	00:24
University/ college degree	05:14	03:52	07:20	03:18	04:30	01:28	00:55	01:18	00:21

At all educational levels, men allocate roughly twice the time devoted by women to SNA work, with the greatest gender difference among the least educated (secondary school not completed). Time devoted to SNA work doubles when women have completed secondary school or above, as compared to women who have not. The most educated men (university/college degree) show the peak SNA working times (7:20 hours).

Unpaid care work does not seem to vary greatly with educational achievement, only slightly decreasing among the more educated men. The opposite seems to occur with care of persons, which increases with education, particularly among the most educated women (university/college degree). This suggests that components of unpaid care work other than care of persons might decrease as educational credentials increase.

As expected, SNA work is marginal for those not in the labour market, and is less than an hour among those who are unemployed. The fact that there is any SNA work for these groups is not necessarily an inconsistency, since the reference period for the labour market status (the previous week) was not the same as the reference period for the activity report (the previous day)[6]. Among those who are employed, women devote almost five hours to SNA work (4:52) and men almost seven hours (6:48).

Those not employed (either unemployed or not in the labour force) devote the longest hours to unpaid care work, particularly women who devote well over five hours to these activities. The greatest gender difference emerges among those who are not in the labour force (40 per cent of women and 19 per cent of men between 15 and 74 years of age), with women devoting 5:15 hours a day to unpaid care work and men 1:46 hours. However, employed women do substantial amounts of unpaid work (three and a half hours) and there is almost no difference in the amount of care of persons that women do whatever their labour market status. Men do more care of persons if

Table 8.3 Mean Time Spent in SNA Work, Unpaid Care Work and Care of Persons, by Sex and Labour Market Status

	SNA work			Unpaid care work			Care of persons		
	Total	Women	Men	Total	Women	Men	Total	Women	Men
Total	03:52	02:45	05:14	03:04	04:18	01:33	00:41	00:58	00:22
Employed	05:53	04:52	06:48	02:24	03:29	01:25	00:39	00:57	00:24
Unemployed	00:50	00:56	00:41	04:26	05:37	02:54	01:02	01:07	00:55
Not in the labour market	00:05	00:04	00:05	04:17	05:15	01:46	00:43	00:58	00:04

they are unemployed (but unemployed men are only 5 per cent of all men between the ages of 15 and 74) and they do almost none if they are not in the labour force (Table 8.3).

As expected given the definition of household headship previously noted, both women and men household heads tend to do more SNA work than non-heads; women who are heads of household work for pay for almost four hours, while men work over six hours. The very few men who are spouses/partners work for pay for roughly the same amount of time (5:59 hours). Women who are spouses/partners work for pay for two hours (2:06) on average. They are the ones who allocate the most time to unpaid care work activities (5:28); and to care of persons (1:18). Men who are household heads devote slightly more time than average both to unpaid care work and to care of persons (Table 8.4).

Turning to the analysis of women's and men's time use patterns according to their household characteristics, we start with the analysis of time use patterns by sex and household types–selected to act as a proxy of relative care burdens that individuals face. Women and men living alone (in one-person households) are the ones who work for pay the most (4:30 hours and 5:34 respectively) and do unpaid care work the least. As care of persons has been defined as care devoted to own household members, it is to be expected that they record almost no time for care of persons.[7].

Although men who live alone are the ones who work for pay the most (5:34 hours), there is only a marginal difference between them and men living in complete nuclear families with children (5:27). Women who do not live alone work for pay the longest when they live in one-parent households (their SNA work reaches almost four hours) and show the longest total

Table 8.4 Mean Time Spent in SNA Work, Unpaid Care Work and Care of Persons, by Sex and Position in Household

	SNA work			Unpaid care work			Care of persons		
	Total	Women	Men	Total	Women	Men	Total	Women	Men
Total	03:52	02:45	05:14	03:04	04:18	01:33	00:41	00:58	00:22
Head of household	05:24	03:57	06:14	02:30	03:43	01:47	00:32	00:42	00:26
Spouse or partner (*)	02:13	02:06	05:59	05:21	05:28	01:21	01:17	01:18	00:21
Daughter/son	02:20	02:00	02:31	01:10	01:33	00:56	00:12	00:17	00:10
Other	03:31	03:04	04:14	02:17	02:54	01:19	00:33	00:43	00:18

*Less than 2 percent of total male population

Table 8.5 Mean Time Spent in SNA Work, Unpaid Care Work and Care of Persons, by Sex and Type of Household

	SNA work			Unpaid care work			Care of persons		
	Total	Women	Men	Total	Women	Men	Total	Women	Men
Total	03:52	02:45	05:14	03:04	04:18	01:33	00:41	00:58	00:22
One person household	04:53	04:30	05:34	02:06	02:22	01:38	00:01	00:00	00:04
Couple without children	03:39	02:31	04:47	02:43	03:44	01:40	00:03	00:58	00:02
Complete nuclear family (with children)	03:43	02:09	05:27	03:33	05:16	01:40	01:06	01:34	00:36
One parent	04:04	03:57	04:18	02:58	03:56	01:10	00:28	00:38	00:09
Extended	03:38	02:27	05:13	03:25	04:41	01:44	00:55	01:17	00:26
Other	03:53	02:25	05:35	01:47	02:44	00:41	00:18	00:34	00:00

*4 percent of total male population

working times: when SNA work is added to unpaid care work, their mean working time reaches almost eight hours (7:53).

Men do more or less the same amount of unpaid care work irrespective of the household type except for the marginal category "in other households"; but they care for persons particularly when they live in complete nuclear families with children. In these families, women's person care time also reaches its peak (1:34 hours).

In terms of SNA work, unpaid care work and care of persons, women and men who live in extended households show patterns that are quite similar to those of women and men living in complete nuclear families.

The presence of children, particularly children aged 5 years or under, makes mean total working times (SNA work plus unpaid care work) reach nearly nine hours a day both for women (8:59 hours) and for men (8:49 hours). Curiously, men's average SNA working time equals women's time for unpaid care work, and the reverse is also true (men's average unpaid care work almost equals women's SNA work). Even if time spent on care of persons is highest among women (3:23 hours) and among men (1:26) when there are children 5 years or under in the household, unpaid care working times far exceed care of persons (which comprises childcare and

Table 8.6 Mean Time Spent in SNA Work, Unpaid Care Work and Care of Persons, by Sex and Presence of Children in Household (24-hour Time)

	SNA work			Unpaid care work			Care of persons		
	Total	Women	Men	Total	Women	Men	Total	Women	Men
Total	03:52	02:45	05:14	03:04	04:18	01:33	00:41	00:58	00:22
In household with . . .									
. . . at least one child 5 or under	04:11	02:32	06:27	02:43	04:44	02:22	02:34	03:32	01:26
. . . children between 6 and 13	03:53	02:19	05:58	03:33	03:50	01:40	01:13	01:39	00:39
. . . adolescents (14–17)	02:46	01:58	03:56	02:58	02:38	01:23	00:15	00:24	00:03
. . . no children or adolescents	04:00	03:07	04:59	03:25	02:29	01:21	00:06	00:07	00:04

Note: There is no overlap between the categories "households with at least one child 5 or under," "households with children 6–13" and "households with only adolescents (14–17)."

elder care), suggesting that children require much more than 'direct' care (Table 8.6)

Women work the most for pay when there are no household members below 18, but they do the same amount of unpaid care work that women in households with only adolescents do, which suggests that the extra burden children impose tends to disappear when children become adolescents (14 to 17 years of age). This is also true about time spent on care of persons.

As households' absolute poverty is related to unemployment and low incomes earned by those who are in the labour market, it is not surprising that average SNA work differs substantially between women and men living in poor and non-poor households. As income is also an indicator of the relative ability to purchase market substitutes for unpaid care work and care services, it is also not surprising that mean time spent on unpaid care work and care of persons in poor households exceeds—and far exceeds in the case of women—the time of those in non-poor households (Table 8.7). Demographic aspects—the greater presence of children and lower incidence of one-person households among poor households—could also be part of

Table 8.7 Mean Time Spent in SNA Work, Unpaid Care Work and Care of Persons, by Sex and Household Absolute Poverty (24-hour time)

	SNA work			Unpaid care work			Care of persons		
	Total	Women	Men	Total	Women	Men	Total	Women	Men
Total	03:58	02:49	05:25	03:09	04:23	01:35	00:44	01:01	00:22
Poor household	01:48	00:59	02:55	04:23	06:14	01:50	01:36	02:27	00:26
Non-poor household	04:08	02:58	05:36	03:03	04:14	01:34	00:39	00:54	00:21

Note: All figures based on a sample of individuals whose households provided complete answers to question/s on total family income.

the explanation for these patterns. The multivariate analysis presented later in this chapter will help disentangle the different contributing factors.

Mean population times devoted to SNA work, unpaid care work and care of persons result from the combined effect of rates of participation and mean times per participant, since mean population times average the time of both participants' times and those who do not perform the activity. But these aggregate figures, though informative, say nothing about the relative burden that those who participate in different types of work shoulder. Indeed, many questions were left unanswered by the previous analysis: Is it that women are more likely to work for pay as household income increases/ children grow? Or is it that they all participate but in varying degrees/hours of paid work? Who are the ones who engage in care for persons the most? Are women/men who live in households with greater care needs equally likely to shoulder them?

Following the structure of Table 8.1 through Table 8.7, the analysis turns now to participation rates, differentiating SNA work, unpaid care work and care of persons.

Rates of participation in SNA work stand at 36 per cent among women and 58 per cent among men. They are somewhat lower than labour market participation rates that emerge from the Annual Household Survey for the population 15 to 74 years (55 per cent among women, 76 per cent among men), since time-use estimations for the "average" day include weekends, holidays, paid leave, etc.

Men's and women's participation rates in SNA work differ substantially by age. While participation rates for young people (15–24) of both sexes are comparable (21 per cent in the case of women and 26 per cent in the case of men), the participation rate in SNA work reaches its peak for women between the ages of 25 and 39 (48 per cent), then declines throughout the following age brackets until retirement age to around 40 per cent. The peak for men, on the other hand, is in the 40–49 bracket, when participation reaches 83 per cent.

Participation rates in unpaid care work are very high for both women and men, since 94 per cent of women and 72 per cent of men devote at least some time to unpaid care work. Participation rates rise with age for both men and women, and are 90 per cent or higher among women above the age of 24. Men also undertake unpaid care work, but to a lesser extent. Men in the 25–39 age bracket and those above retirement age are the ones who participate in unpaid care work the most (81 per cent and 85 per cent respectively).

Only 30 per cent of women and 20 per cent of men take part in care of persons. Peak ages for participation in care of persons coincide with peak ages of participation in SNA work. Fifty-seven per cent of women 25–39 participate, while for men between the ages of 40 and 49, this figure reaches its peak at 41 per cent. This age perspective must be supplemented by household life-cycle indicators, as will be done in the following paragraph.

The rate of participation in paid work rises with educational levels, for both men and women. Twenty-eight per cent of women and 58 per cent of men who have not completed secondary school engage in paid work, as compared to 46 per cent and 74 per cent of women and men who have completed a university/tertiary degree. This is expected as earnings tend to increase with educational achievement. Among women, there are no substantial differences in participation in unpaid care work with educational levels; though the most highly educated women participate proportionally more in care of persons (38 per cent). Quite the opposite, men do not show striking differences in their participation in care of persons according to their educational levels; but the most involved in unpaid care work are the most educated men (80 per cent).

SNA work performed by those who are not in the labour force is marginal also in terms of participation rates. The unemployed, though few in number, seem to be more engaged in SNA work than expected, particularly men (18 per cent).

Women undertake unpaid care work in slightly higher proportions when they are not in the labour force (96 per cent), though this is not related to higher participation in care of persons. Indeed, women who are employed participate more than their inactive counterparts in care of persons (32 per cent and 28 per cent, respectively). This would suggest that actor time moves in the opposite direction, to make mean times similar (Table 8.3). Men are more likely to engage in unpaid care work (75 per cent) and care of persons (23 per cent) when they are employed.

Male and female heads of household participate more in SNA work than do other household members of the same sex (68 per cent and 48 per cent, respectively), and less in unpaid care work and care of persons than spouses/partners, thus highlighting the time pressure that breadwinning responsibility creates for heads of household and the correspondingly reduced time available for providing care.

In general terms, heads of household and spouses/partners are more likely to participate in unpaid care work (93 per cent and 98 per cent respectively among women, 78 per cent and 89 per cent among men) than daughters/sons and other household members of the same sex, though gender differences in participation are present among all member types. The same pattern is also true for participation rates of daughters/sons and other members in care of persons.

The type of household seems to be a major factor determining participation in SNA work, unpaid care work and care of persons. Showing a similar pattern to that for mean population times, members of one-person households participate the most in SNA work (57 per cent), and the least in care of persons (2 per cent), as might be expected in the absence of a household care burden. In addition, the participation of these men and women in unpaid care work (comprised in this case of household maintenance and unpaid community services) are similar (86 per cent), but show the striking feature that women who live alone participate the least in unpaid care work among women, while among men, those who live alone participate the most. Indeed, unpaid care work clearly shifts from men to women as household size increases. At the extreme, only 68 per cent of men living in extended households undertake unpaid care work.

The women who are most likely to participate in care of persons are those living in extended-family households (50 per cent). In addition, participation in care of persons is very high among both men and women in complete nuclear families with children (32 per cent and 45 per cent, respectively). As opposed to men, women in one-parent households show relatively high participation rates in care of persons (27 per cent).

The presence of children and their age are related to the phase of the life cycle that women's and men's households are going through. Women with no children in their households are the ones who engage in SNA work the most (38 per cent) and in care of persons the least (5 per cent), as it was the case with their mean working times.

Women's rate of participation in SNA work in households with young children or pre-adolescents is high—indeed, close to the average—declining only in households with adolescents. This is due in part to the fact that adolescents themselves were among the survey's informants, and their rate of participation in paid work is very low.

The presence and age of children in the household is associated with men's participation in unpaid care work and in care of persons: men's participation rates reach 84 per cent and 72 per cent respectively when there is at least one child aged 5 years or under in the household. Almost all women (91 per cent) who live in households where there are children 5 or under undertake care of persons irrespective of their age and their relationship to the household head. Both women's and men's participation rates in care of persons decline markedly as the age of the youngest child in the household increases. This indicates that despite clear gender differences, the enormous care needs of young children require great involvement on the part of both women and men.

Differences in mean population times according to the household economic situation—already shown in Table 8.7—are clearly related to differences in participation rates, which are particularly striking in SNA work and care of persons. Women and men who live in non-poor households show participation rates in SNA work (38 per cent and 62 per cent) which are double those of women and men living in poor households. In turn, poor women's and men's participation rates in care of persons (69 per cent and 36 per cent) are more than double those of non-poor women and men. Differences in unpaid care work are less marked, with non-poor men participating slightly more than poor men and the opposite happening among women.

EXPLORING CARE OF PERSONS IN MORE DETAIL

Having analysed both mean population times and participation rates in care of persons, in this section the focus turns to the time that is allocated to care of persons per participant or "actor" i.e. the time spent by those who undertook care of persons activities.

A distinctive feature of activities related to care of persons is that even though relatively few people participate, those who participate tend to do so quite extensively; women who participate devote over three hours and men almost two hours to care of persons activities (24-hour time). Table 8.8 shows that gender differences in mean population times result from both differences in participation rates—women participating far more than men—and differences in participants' times—women who participate devoting on average an hour more than men who participate (24-hour time).

The relationship between mean full-minute times and mean 24-hour times spent on an activity or group of activities is known as the simultaneity ratio. The simultaneity ratio for care of persons is roughly 1.32 for women and 1.33 for men. These ratios are among the highest recorded for any activity in Buenos Aires along with leisure time activities and activities involving the use of communications media (Esquivel 2010). The simultaneity ratios for care of persons "expand" mean actor time by one hour among women (from 3:07 hours to 4:07 hours) and by more than half an hour among men (from 1:52 to 2:30). Given these high simultaneity ratios, this section's analysis will focus on full-minute times. For the reader to be able to compare the previous analysis, which was based on 24-hour time, and this section's, all tables show times per actor using both the 24-hour time and the full-minute time. Also, participation rates are repeated in all tables to remind the reader that the analysis refers to times per actor.

Table 8.8 Mean Time Per Actor and Rate of Participation in Care of Persons (%), by Sex and Age

	Women			Men		
	24-hour time per actor	Full-minute time per actor	Participation rate	24-hour time per actor	Full-minute time per actor	Participation rate
Total	03:07	04:07	31	01:52	02:30	20
15 to 24 years	01:47	02:42	20	01:28	02:18	6
25 to 39 years	03:38	04:52	57	02:19	03:02	35
40 to 49 years	03:05	04:12	38	01:29	02:02	41
50 to 64 years	02:25	02:44	19	01:47	02:17	4
65 to 74 years	03:53	04:14	5	00:32	00:35	3

Among women, those who participate more in care of persons are also those who devote more time to these activities: women in the 25 to 39 age bracket devote little less than 5 hours to caring activities (4:52 hours). Young women (15 to 24 years of age) and women just below retirement age (50 to 64 years of age) participate only in 20 per cent of cases; and devote approximately 2:40 hours on average when they participate. Interestingly, older women (those above retirement age) participate only marginally in care of persons, but for extended periods when they do so (4:14 hours) (Table 8.8).

Among men, those who devote longer times per participant are in the 25 to 39 age bracket. Their mean participant time is substantially lower than women's of the same age (three hours), as is their participation rate, which is almost half that of women. Men between 40 and 49 years of age participate in care of persons in over 40 per cent of cases, but devote to these activities below-average times when they participate (2:02 hours).

Person care times for those who participate—whether men or women—increase markedly with education, reaching 4:24 hours among women and 2:48 hours among the most educated men. In the case of women, mean participants' time is also accompanied by higher participation rates, while this is not the case among men.

Mean times per participant are higher among women who are not in the labour market, although their participation is slightly lower than for employed women. Men not in the labour market (who are 19 per cent of all men in the population under scrutiny) tend neither to engage in care of persons nor to devote substantial times when they do (only 7 per cent of them devote on average 1:40 hours). Times dedicated to care of persons are the

Table 8.9 Mean Time Per Actor and Rate of Participation in Care of Persons (%), by Sex and Educational Level

	Women			Men		
	24-hour time per actor	Full-minute time per actor	Participation rate	24-hour time per actor	Full-minute time per actor	Participation rate
Total	03:07	04:07	31	01:52	02:30	20
Secondary not completed	02:56	03:52	26	01:42	02:22	18
Secondary completed/ university not completed	03:01	04:03	29	01:55	02:27	22
University/ college degree	00:24	04:24	38	01:59	02:48	18

Table 8.10 Mean Time Per Actor and Participation Rate in Care of Persons (%), by Sex and Labour Market Status

	Women			Men		
	24-hour time per actor	Full-minute time per actor	Participation rate	24-hour time per actor	Full-minute time per actor	Participation rate
Total	03:07	04:07	31	01:52	02:30	20
Employed	02:58	03:53	32	01:46	02:21	23
Unemployed	02:41	03:58	41	05:57	08:01	16
Not in the labour market	03:29	04:32	28	01:04	01:40	7

*Less than 5 percent of total population

highest among unemployed participants, both women and men. However, given their small numbers they will not be analysed[8].

It is among female spouses—who are the women with the highest participation rate—that time devoted to care of persons is the longest, reaching 4:31 hours, which is half an hour more than the average for women. The female heads of household who participate in care of persons (one quarter of them) devote 3:40 hours to these activities. Among men, it is sons and other members who devote the longest times to care, although their participation rates are quite low and participants amount to only 30 per cent of the male population (Table 8.11). One quarter of male household heads participate in care of persons and devote 2:21 hours on average to these activities.

Very low participation rates among women and men living in households that account for small fractions of the population (one-person households plus couples without children account for 25 per cent of total population) impede detailed analysis. Focusing on the population living in nuclear families, one-parent households and extended households (67 per cent of total population) two features emerge: the high participation rates that accompany high time allocation per participant among women; and men's mean times per actor being lower and less variable than those of women.

In particular, half of women living in extended families devote almost three hours on average to care of persons, while almost half of women (45 per cent) living in complete nuclear families with children devote nearly five hours (4:45) to care of persons. In this case, it is the combination of above average participation rates and long time allocation per actor which

Table 8.11 Mean Time Per Actor and Rate of Participation in Care of Persons (%), by Sex and Position in Household

	Women			Men		
	24-hour time per actor	Full-minute time per actor	Participation rate	24-hour time per actor	Full-minute time per actor	Participation rate
Total	03:07	04:07	31	01:52	02:30	20
Head of household	02:53	03:40	25	01:48	02:21	24
Spouse or partner (*)	03:21	04:31	39	01:07	01:19	32
Daughter/son	01:53	02:25	15	02:40	04:26	7
Other	02:50	03:22	25	02:06	02:43	14

*Less than 2 percent of total male population

Table 8.12 Mean Time Per Actor and Rate of Participation in Care of Persons (%), by Sex and Type of Household

	Women			Men		
	24-hour time per actor	Full-minute time per actor	Participation rate	24-hour time per actor	Full-minute time per actor	Participation rate
Total	03:07	04:07	31	01:52	02:30	20
One person household			0	01:45	02:04	4
Couple without children	00:02	02:52	4	01:19	01:22	3
Complete nuclear family (with children)	03:28	04:45	45	01:52	02:32	32
One parent	02:24	03:07	27	01:58	02:51	8
Extended	02:33	02:57	50	02:06	02:45	21
Other	03:04	03:32	19	00:21	00:30	2

*4 percent of the total population

explains higher than average figures in Table 8.5 and supports the idea that it is precisely in these households that the care burden is greatest.

Mean actor time devoted to care of persons, as well as participation rates, are highly correlated with the presence of children, and decrease as the age of the child or children increases. Amounts peak at 5:06 hours among women and 2:33 among men living in households with at least one child 5 years old or under. As it was noted previously, it is in these households that the rate of participation in care of persons is also the highest (91 per cent for women and 72 per cent for men), suggesting that the main driver of care of persons is children and not care for adults. The difference between the time devoted by participating men and participating women (approximately 50 per cent) persists as childcare needs decrease with children's increasing age (Table 8.13).

Figures in Table 8.14 emphasise what was already said when analysing participation rates in care of persons. Indeed, seven out of ten poor women devote 5 hours on average to care of persons, while only one third of women in non-poor households engage in care of persons, devoting four hours to it. Relatively similar mean population times for poor and non-poor men shown in Table 8.7 are a combination of lower participation rates and slightly higher mean participants' times for non-poor men; and participation rates that almost double the average participation rate for men but lower times per participant among poor men.

Table 8.13 Mean Time Per Actor and Participation Rate in Care of Persons (%), by Sex and Presence of Children in Household

	Women			Men		
	24-hour time per actor	Full-minute time per actor	Participation rate	24-hour time per actor	Full-minute time per actor	Participation rate
Total	03:07	04:07	31	01:52	02:30	20
In households with ...						
... at least one child age 5 or under	03:44	05:06	91	02:01	02:33	72
... children between 6 and 13	02:41	03:25	62	01:35	02:14	41
... adolescents (14–17)	01:49	02:03	22	00:39	00:53	9
... neither children or adolescents (*)	02:22	02:50	5	02:29	04:00	3

Note: There is no overlap between the categories "households with at least one child 5 or under," "households with children 6–13" and "households with only adolescents (14–17)."
* Special cases: fathers and mothers who do not live with their children most of the week, thus their children are technically not members of their households. For an explanation of this and other methodological features of the Buenos Aires TUS, see Esquivel (2010).

Table 8.14 Mean Time Per Actor and Participation Rate in Care of Persons (%), by Sex and Household Absolute Poverty

	Women			Men		
	24-hour time per actor	Full-minute time per actor	Participation rate	24-hour time per actor	Full-minute time per actor	Participation rate
Total	03:11	04:12	32	01:50	02:32	20
Poor	03:33	04:59	69	01:13	02:01	36
Non-poor	03:07	04:03	29	01:55	02:36	19

Note: All figures based on a sample of individuals whose households provided complete answers to question/s on total family income.

MULTIVARIATE ANALYSIS OF KEY DETERMINANTS OF CARE TIME

How do each of the factors analysed above impact on the time that is devoted to unpaid care work and care of persons? The following are marginal effects (valued at the mean of included variables[9]) resulting from two pairs of Tobit regressions of the full-minute time (expressed in minutes per day) devoted to unpaid care work (Table 8.15) and care of persons (Table 8.16) by men and women.

Descriptive analysis has shown that women and men have different participation times, and times per actor in unpaid care work and care of persons. Splitting regression analysis by sex makes it possible to analyse the covariates that explain women's and men's unpaid productive time, and show their differential statistical significance and their relative influence on women and men.

Regressions in Table 8.15 are run on the whole sample (593 men and 815 women), while regressions in Table 8.16 are run excluding one-person households (485 men and 637 women). Restricting the sample for the analysis of care of persons to households in which there are persons to be cared for guarantees that zero values are indeed associated with non-participation. The exception is the aforementioned "special cases" in which fathers and mothers of children who do not live with them during most of the week devote time to childcare on the surveyed day. These six cases are recorded as one-parent households; otherwise, they would have been (incorrectly) excluded from the analysis.

All covariates analysed in the previous descriptive sections are included in regressions for women and men. Instead of presence of children, the number of household's children in each age threshold (5 or under; between 6 and 13; between 14 and 17) is used, as marginal effects are more clearly read using this specification. In the case of parents of non living-in children, the number of living-in children is zero.

It is interesting to contrast first men's and women's estimated participation probabilities for unpaid care work and care of persons in Table 8.15 and Table 8.16. Consistent with descriptive analysis, the estimated probability of participation in unpaid care work is much higher than that of care of persons; and higher for women (96 per cent) than for men (74 per cent). Gender differences in estimated participation also are evident in care of persons, as women's estimated participation (45 per cent) almost doubles that of men's (23 per cent).

Turning first to unpaid care work as a whole, both women's and men's daily time devoted to these activities is inversely related to employment status. For both women and men, age is positively associated with unpaid care work (at a decreasing rate); though the number and ages of household children is the strongest determinant. One more pre-school child increases women's unpaid care work by almost two and a half hours and men's unpaid

Table 8.15 Marginal Effects for Tobit Conditional on Positive Unpaid Care Work, by Sex

	Men			Women		
	Coefficient	Sig.	Mean	Coefficient	Sig.	Mean
Household head	-2.0		0.76	84.4	***	0.42
Spouse/partner	-10.2		0.02	126.7	***	0.42
Daughter/son	-26.3		0.17	-65.4	*	0.09
Employed	-66.0	***	0.77	-133.2	***	0.58
Secondary comp./tertiary not completed	13.0		0.44	-24.8		0.41
Tertiary/college degree	10.8		0.23	-26.0		0.29
Age	7.0	***	42.1	13.5	***	44.7
Square of the 'age' mean	-0.1	***	1770.7	-0.1	***	1996.9
Number of children < 6 years	68.2	***	0.20	143.6	***	0.22
Number of children 6–13 years	21.0	**	0.28	36.2	***	0.31
Number of children 14–17 years	-0.9		0.17	-19.2		0.18
Couple without children (*)	-2.1		0.16	35.4		0.14
Complete nuclear family with children (*)	-32.9	**	0.41	108.6	***	0.34
One-parent household (*)	34.8		0.10	122.9	***	0.13
Extended household (*)	-25.5		0.09	49.3		0.09
Other households (*)	-49.6	***	0.07	108.7	***	0.08
Poor (*)	0.8		0.06	94.3	***	0.07
Scale factor used for marginal effects	0.53			0.83		
Estimated participation probability	0.74			0.96		
Rho2	0.15			0.43		
N	593			815		

Note: Statistically significant to 99 per cent***; 95 per cent**; 90 per cent*.
* marginal effect dy/dx is for discrete change of dummy variable from 0 to 1
Base case: other household members; not employed; secondary not completed; no children in the household; one-person household; non-poor household.

care work by over an hour a day. The impact of an "extra" school-age child is much weaker. The number of adolescents is not significant in either case.

Women who participate in this work devote longer times to unpaid care work than the base case when they live in nuclear households with children; and when they live in more complex ("other") households (108 minutes more in both cases). Men, on the other hand, spend between half an hour and 49 minutes *less* than the base case when they live in the very same household types. Women living in one-parent households devote over 2 hours more to unpaid care work than the base case.

For women, being a household head or spouse/partner is also strongly and positively associated with unpaid care work time; while being a daughter is an hour a day less demanding as compared to the base case ("other" household members). In contrast, men's unpaid care work is not affected by their position in the household.

As opposed to findings in previous descriptive sections, educational attainment is neither related to unpaid care work nor to care of persons—i.e. other covariates explain those findings.

Children remain among the strongest determinants of women's and men's care of persons. One more pre-school age child make women caregivers provide an hour and a half more care than in the base case; while school-age children result in half an hour more. Results are less strong for men, yet significant in statistical terms: men who participate in care of persons devote three quarters of an hour for every "extra" pre-school age child; and 21 minutes for every school-age child.

As opposed to unpaid care work as a whole, household types are significant and positively associated to men's care of persons, as compared to the base case (couples without children). In particular, men who live in one-parent households (single/divorced parents or sons) devote almost three hours to care of persons when they participate. The same household effect is present among women. This suggests that household type influences the time dedicated to care beyond the individual's position in the household. Note also that the presence of adolescents reduces men's time spent on care of persons.

Women living in poor households devote an hour and a half more time than those in non-poor households to unpaid care work, and half an hour more to care of persons (conditional on participating); but, contrary to descriptive findings, there is no difference for men related to their household's poverty status. This might be an indication that it is women's time, but not men's time, that adjusts in order to counterbalance low household income. Absolute poverty is related to longer women's care times either because there is little possibility for purchasing care substitutes and/or because absolute poverty is also related to restricted access to care facilities provided by the state or the community. Regrettably, regression analysis does not tell whether the fact that the poor women do more unpaid care work and more care of persons is a result of the existence of worse opportunities for income-earning work, or the cause of them.

Table 8.16 Marginal Effects for Tobit Conditional on Positive Care of Persons, by Sex

	Men			Women		
	Coffecient	Sig.	Mean	Coffecient	Sig.	Mean
Household head	18.9		0.71	53.7	**	0.27
Spouse/partner	21.9		0.03	48.2	**	0.54
Daughter/son	-40.3	*	0.20	-31.5		0.11
Employed	-9.6		0.78	-15.5		0.56
Secondary comp./tertiary not completed	-6.9		0.41	-0.4		0.40
Tertiary/college degree	-13.8		0.23	5.0		0.28
Age	7.2	**	41.6	1.6		43.0
Square of the 'age' mean	-0.1	***	1729.4	0.0		1851.2
Number of children < 6 years	44.5	***	0.25	88.6	***	0.28
Number of children 6–13 years	21.7	***	0.34	33.2	***	0.40
Number of children 14–17 years	-8.2	***	0.21	-7.0		0.23
Nuclear family with children	44.8	**	0.50	64.7	***	0.43
One-parent household (*)	169.0	***	0.12	70.1	***	0.43
Extended household (*)	66.1	**	0.11	51.6	**	0.11
Other households (*)	-5.5		0.08	85.6	**	0.10
Poor (*)	0.2		0.07	28.5	*	0.09
Scale factor used for marginal effects	0.23			0.34		
Estimated participation probability	0.23			0.45		
$Rho2$	0.19			0.40		
N	485			637		

Note: Statistically significant to 99 per cent***; 95 per cent**; 90 per cent*.
* marginal effect dy/dx is for discrete change of dummy variable from 0 to 1
Base case: other household members; not employed; secondary not completed; no children in the household; one-person household; non-poor household.

Multivariate analysis reveals that times devoted to unpaid care work are highly sensitive to gender, employment status, and the number and age of household's children. Women's household position (relative to the head of household); the household structure and household incomes below the poverty line also determine women's unpaid care work.

Except for employment status, the same picture emerges in the analysis of care of persons. However, men's care of persons seems to be more responsive than their unpaid care work to household burdens, as indicated by the statistical significance of the number of pre-school age and school age children and household structure.

In sum, multivariate analysis confirms main descriptive analysis findings, only strongly rejecting any role for education in determining participation rates and times devoted to unpaid care work and care of persons.

SUMMARISING MAIN FINDINGS: UNPAID CARE WORK IN THE CITY OF BUENOS AIRES

Generally speaking, the preceding results are not surprising. They show the entrenched gender differences in the distribution of unpaid care work, a work that requires time and energy but does not generate an income for those who perform it. This is the first time, though, that these differences can be measured in the Argentine context and the questions "how much care work is performed in the City of Buenos Aires?" and "who performs it?" receive concrete (and methodologically sound) answers.

There are also some surprising results. For example, the fact that women's and men's population mean times devoted to total work do not differ much—only 15 minutes—is somewhat unexpected. Women and men who work more (SNA work plus unpaid care work) are the employed; heads of households; those with children aged 5 or under living in the household and women living in one-parent households.

Substantial gender differences emerge in the distribution of working time within different types of work, and for different population subgroups. While SNA work is only one third of women's total work, income-generating activities represent three quarters of all men's work. These gender differences are associated with women participating less in the labour market than men, and not with shorter hours of paid work for those who are employed (DGEyC, 2007c). They are also associated with the fact that unpaid care work is mostly performed by women. As an illustration of the latter, women and men who live alone are equally likely to do at least some unpaid care work in an average day, but this level of participation in unpaid care work of 86 per cent is the highest among men and the lowest among women across different types of households. As households and families gain in complexity, and care requirements rise accordingly, unpaid care work participation and times shift from men to women.

In contrast with more traditional patterns found in other developing countries, men in the City of Buenos Aires engage in care of persons, particularly those with pre-school age and school age children, even if the time they devote to care of persons is substantially less than the time devoted by women who participate. Patterns of care of persons are not exactly like those of developed countries either, since poor women perform more person care. Multivariate analysis has indeed confirmed that households' income poverty combines with—and possibly reinforces–gender inequality in the distribution of unpaid care work and care of persons.

Results have shed light on the extent and nature of "invisible" gender inequalities that are at the root of the more visible unequal distribution of resources and opportunities among men and women in the City of Buenos Aires.

NOTES

1. See the Buenos Aires Time Use Survey webpage. http://www.buenosaires.gov.ar/hacienda/sis_estadistico/eah_2005.php?menu_id=22670, accessed August 2008.
2. Those living in boarding houses and shanty towns have been excluded. See DGEyC (2005b).
3. Since the survey question uses the traditional masculine gender in asking who is head of household ("Please tell me all of the people making up this household, starting with *el jefe*," i.e. "the [male] head"), and since head of household status is associated with power, as is masculinity, it is not frequent for a woman to designate herself as the head of household of a complete nuclear family, even when she earns more than her husband (unless he is unemployed or not in the labour market).
4. Paid domestic workers are regarded as members of the household they work for if they live-in most of the week.
5. Corresponding coefficients of variation have been published in DGEyC (2007c).
6. The Buenos Aires Time Use Survey was not designed to improve on the Annual Household Survey's ability to capture SNA work data, as the latter coincide with the Buenos Aires data from the Current Household Survey used to calculate national unemployment figures. See Esquivel (2010) for a detailed review of the Buenos Aires Time Use Survey objectives.
7. In fact they should devote none. Recorded times are the result of a handful of sample "special cases." See the following.
8. The fact that the group of unemployed caregivers is very small when compared to the total population (1.9 per cent of women and 0.7 per cent of men) means that the figure of 8 hours recorded for male caregivers is not reliable.
9. Strictly speaking, results are valued at regressors' means except for the square of the age mean (instead of the mean of age squared). For details on Tobit, see Wooldrige (2002).

REFERENCES

Budlender, Debbie. 2007. *A Critical Review of Selected Time Use Surveys*. Gender and Development Programme Paper No. 2. UNRISD, Geneva.

Dirección General de Estadística y Censos, Ciudad Autónoma de Buenos Aires (DGEyC). 2005a. Encuesta de Uso del Tiempo 2005. Clasificador de Actividades, Buenos Aires. http://estatico.buenosaires.gov.ar/areas/hacienda/sis_estadistico/2005/clasificador_actividades.pdf, accessed August 2008.

Dirección General de Estadística y Censos, Ciudad Autónoma de Buenos Aires (DGEyC). 2005b. Síntesis metodológica Encuesta de Uso del Tiempo 2005, Buenos Aires. http://estatico.buenosaires.gov.ar/areas/hacienda/sis_estadistico/2005/eut_sintesis.pdf, accessed August 2008.

Dirección General de Estadística y Censos, Ciudad Autónoma de Buenos Aires (DGEyC). 2007a. "Encuesta Anual de Hogares 2005, Encuesta de Uso del Tiempo, El tiempo de trabajo total. Mujeres y varones en la Ciudad de Buenos Aires," Informe de Resultados No. 328, September, Buenos Aires. http://buenosaires.gov.ar/areas/hacienda/sis_estadistico/informe_328_encuesta_de_uso_del_tiempo.pdf, accessed August 2008.

Dirección General de Estadística y Censos, Ciudad Autónoma de Buenos Aires (DGEyC). 2007b. "Encuesta Anual de Hogares 2005, Encuesta de Uso del Tiempo, La utilización del tiempo de las mujeres y los varones," Informe de Resultados No. 329, September, Buenos Aires. http://buenosaires.gov.ar/areas/hacienda/sis_estadistico/informe_329_encuesta_de_uso_del_tiempo.pdf, accessed August 2008.

Dirección General de Estadística y Censos, Ciudad Autónoma de Buenos Aires (DGEyC). 2007c. "Encuesta de Uso del Tiempo 2005. Cuadros básicos," Buenos Aires. http://estatico.buenosaires.gov.ar/areas/hacienda/sis_estadistico/2005/eut_cuad_basicos.pdf, accessed August 2008.

Esquivel, Valeria. 2010. "Lessons from the Buenos Aires Time Use Survey. A Methodological Assessment," in Rania Antonopoulos and Indira Hirway, eds. *Unpaid Work and the Economy: Gender, Time Use and Poverty*. Palgrave-Mcmillan, New York.

Esquivel, Valeria. 2008. Time-Use Surveys in Latin America. In Valeria Esquivel, Debbie Budlender, Nancy Folbre and Indira Hirway, "Explorations: Time-use surveys in the South", *Feminist Economics*. Vol. 14, No. 3, July, pp. 107–152.

United Nations Statistics Division (UNSD). 2005. *Guide to Producing Statistics on Time Use: Measuring Paid and Unpaid Work*. Department of Economic and Social Affairs, United Nations, New York.

Wooldrige, Jeffrey. 2002. *Econometric Analysis of Cross Section and Panel Data*. MIT Press, London.

Index

Note: Page numbers followed by 'f' refer to figures and page numbers followed by 't' refer to tables.

24-hour minute 6

A
age: in Buenos Aires time spent on care of persons by sex and 211, 211t, 221; in Buenos Aires time spent on paid and unpaid work by sex and 29, 201–2, 201t, 207–8; combining with gender 29; in India time spent on childcare by sex and 107–8, 108t; in India time spent on SNA and extended SNA by location, sex and 29, 97–8, 97t; in Japan time spent on paid and unpaid work by sex and 144, 144t, 151; in Korea time spent on paid and unpaid work by sex and 29, 126–7, 127t, 139; in Nicaragua time spent on SNA, paid work and unpaid care work by sex and 29, 182–3, 183t, 194; in South Africa time spent on paid and unpaid work by sex and 29, 75–6, 75t, 84; survey age groups 9; in Tanzania time spent on paid and unpaid work by sex and 29, 52, 52t, 59; and Tobit estimations in respect of care of persons 28t, 62, 62t, 85t, 123, 123t, 124t, 125, 148, 149t, 188, 190t; and Tobit estimations in respect of unpaid care work 25, 26t, 62, 63t, 85t, 86, 114t, 115, 115t, 116, 123, 123t, 124t, 125, 188, 189t

Argentina: see Buenos Aires
Australia 10

B
Belgium 153t

Bittman, M. 5, 10, 16
Budig, M. 10, 11
Buenos Aires 197–222; care dependency ratio 33, 33f, 34, 34f; comparison of composition of hours spent on SNA and unpaid care work by country and sex 18, 19, 19f; comparison of mean time spent per day on activities by SNA category, country and sex 15f; comparison of mean time spent per day on activities by SNA category, country and sex for actors 17f; comparison of mean time spent per day on activities by sub-category of unpaid care work, country and sex 21, 22f, 23; comparison of mean time spent per day on sub-categories of unpaid care work by country and sex for actors 23, 23f; comparison of participation rates by SNA category, country and sex 13f, 14; comparison of participation rates by sub-category of unpaid care work, country and sex 20–1, 21f; female economic activity rate and share 11t; methodology for survey 7, 8–9, 8t, 197–8; simultaneous time capture 6, 7; survey population description 198–200; Tobit estimations on care of persons 27, 28t, 216–20, 219t; Tobit estimations on unpaid care work 25, 26t, 216–20, 217t; value of unpaid care work 37, 38, 39f, 41f; see also Buenos Aires care of persons by mean time per

Index

actor and rate of participation; Buenos Aires SNA work, unpaid care work and care of persons

Buenos Aires care of persons by mean time per actor and rate of participation 210–15; by age and sex 211, 211t, 221; by children in household and sex 214, 215t; by educational level and sex 211, 212t; by household absolute poverty and sex 214, 215t; by household position and sex 213, 213t; by household type and sex 213–14, 214t; by labour market status and sex 211, 212t, 213; simultaneity ratio for care of persons 210

Buenos Aires SNA work, unpaid care work and care of persons: by age and sex, mean time spent 29, 201–2, 201t; by age and sex, participation rate 207–8; by children in household and sex, mean time spent 205–6, 206t; by children in household and sex, participation rate 209–10; composition of total working time by sex 200f; by educational level and sex, mean time spent 202t, 203; by educational level and sex, participation rate 208; by household absolute poverty and sex, mean time spent 206–7, 207t; by household absolute poverty and sex, participation rate 210; by household position and sex, mean time spent 204, 204t; by household position and sex, participation rate 208–9; by household type and sex, mean time spent 204–5, 205t, 214; by household type and sex, participation rate 209; by labour market status and sex, mean time spent 29, 203–4, 203t; by labour market status and sex, participation rate 208

C

Canada 15, 43
care dependency ratio 3, 31–4, 33f, 121, 186, 187t
Carrasco, C. 171
caste 97, 100, 108t, 116; and Tobit estimations in respect of care of persons 27, 28t, 115t, 116; and Tobit estimations in respect of unpaid care work 25, 26t, 114t, 115

Central Statistical Organisation 92

childcare: developed countries time spent on 10, 11–12, 22, 153–4, 153t, 168–9; ideological aspects of reporting on 11–12; simultaneous time capture 6; *see also* India and time spent on childcare; Japan and time spent on childcare

children in household: in Buenos Aires time spent on care of persons by sex and 214, 215t; in Buenos Aires time spent on paid and unpaid work by sex and 205–6, 206t, 209–10; gender combined with 29–30; in India time spent on paid and unpaid work by sex, location and 29–30, 99–100, 99t; in Japan time spent on paid and unpaid work by sex and 30, 144, 145t, 146, 151, 152; in Korea time spent on paid and unpaid work by sex and 129–30, 131t, 140; in Nicaragua time spent on SNA, paid work and unpaid care work by sex and 30, 184–5, 185t, 194; in South Africa time spent on paid and unpaid work by sex and 30, 76–7, 77t, 84; in Tanzania time spent on paid and unpaid work by sex and 53t, 54, 59; and Tobit estimations in respect of care of persons 25, 27, 28t, 61, 62t, 85, 85t, 123, 123t, 124t, 125, 148, 149t, 188, 190t; and Tobit estimations in respect of childcare 150, 150t, 151; and Tobit estimations in respect of unpaid care work 62, 63t, 85t, 86, 114t, 115, 115t, 116, 123, 123t, 124t, 125, 147t, 148, 188, 189t

City of Buenos Aires' Annual Household Survey 197

classifications for unpaid work 4–5

community service 20, 21, 21f, 22–3, 22f, 113–14

Craig, L. 10

D

Denmark 18

developed countries: care of persons, time spent on 22; childcare, time spent on 10, 11–12, 22, 153–4, 153t, 168–9; and differences with studies in developing countries xxi–xxii, 10–12, 22; division of time between SNA and non-SNA activities 18; focus on studies in 1; and gender divisions between SNA and extended-SNA 10, 14; influence of education on time spent on unpaid care work 25; Pacholok and Gauthier's study of paid and unpaid work patterns in 15, 25, 43

diary approach to time recording 5–6

domestic workers: approach to calculating value of unpaid care work 37, 39, 137t, 140; employed in home 54, 78, 79, 102, 194

E

earnings, approaches to measuring 35–6

Economically Active Population Survey of NSO 135–6, 138

education: in Buenos Aires time spent on care of persons by sex and 211, 212t; in Buenos Aires time spent on paid and unpaid work by sex and 202t, 203, 208; in India time spent on childcare by economic variables and 109, 110t; in India time spent on SNA and extended SNA by location, sex and 100, 101t; influence on women's engagement with unpaid care work 25; in Korea time spent on paid and unpaid work by sex and 127–9, 128t, 139–40; in Tanzania time spent on paid and unpaid work by sex and 55t, 56, 61; and Tobit estimations in respect of care of persons 27, 28t, 61, 62t, 85t, 123, 123t, 124, 124t, 148, 149t; and Tobit estimations in respect of childcare 150–1, 150t; and Tobit estimations in respect of unpaid care work 25, 26t, 62, 63t, 85t, 86, 114t, 115, 115t, 116, 123, 123t, 124t, 125, 147t, 148

elderly care: and care of sick and disabled in India 106–7, 106t; and Tobit estimations in respect of 147t, 148, 149t, 169; *see also* Japan and time spent on care for elderly

Elson, D. 1, 10, 11

employment: *see* work status

Esquivel, V. 37, 197, 210, 215

Estonia 153t

F

feminist economics xxi, 1, 171

Finland 22, 153t

Folbre, N. 10, 11

France 153t

Franzoni, J. 12

fuel and water collection 5, 31; in Nicaragua 13, 179t; in South Africa 72; in Tanzania 48–9

full minute 6–7

G

Gauthier, A. 15, 25, 43

gender patterns, basic 3, 9–23, 42–4; age combined with 29; children in household combined with 29–30; combined with other influential factors 3, 27–31, 43; comparison of composition of hours spent on SNA and unpaid care work by country and sex 17–19, 19f; comparison of mean time spent per day by on activities by sub-category of unpaid care work, country and sex 21–3, 22f; comparison of mean time spent per day on activities by SNA category, country and sex 14–16, 15f; comparison of mean time spent per day on activities by SNA category, country and sex for actors 16–17, 17f; comparison of mean time spent per day on sub-categories of unpaid care work by country and sex for actors 23, 23f; comparison of participation by sub-category of unpaid care work, country and sex 20–1, 21f; comparison of participation rates by SNA category, country and sex 12–14, 13f; cross-country comparisons 12; developed countries division between SNA and extended SNA

10, 14; Elson's study of change in female share of paid employment 1980–97 10, 11; employment combined with 30–1; and extended SNA 19–23; extended SNA unpaid care work 19–23; female economic activity rate and share 10–12, 11t; Pacholok and Gauthier's research on 15, 43–4; research focus on developed countries 10; SNA-related categories 12–19; and Tobit estimations in respect of care of persons 25, 27, 28t, 61, 62t, 85, 85t, 115t, 116, 123, 123t, 124–5, 124t, 148, 149t, 168; and Tobit estimations in respect of unpaid care work 26t, 62, 63t, 85t, 86, 114t, 115, 123, 123t, 124t, 125, 147t, 148, 168, 188, 189t, 195; UNDP study of division of work time 18

Germany 15, 43, 153t

government expenditure on social services and comparison with value of unpaid care work: in Korea 138, 141; in Nicaragua 193; in South Africa 89–90; in Tanzania 67

Gross Domestic Product: Buenos Aires value of unpaid care work and care of persons as a percentage of 38, 39f; comparisons of value of unpaid care work and care of persons by country as a percentage of 38–40; Indian value of unpaid care work and care of persons as a percentage of 39, 39f; Japanese value of unpaid care work and care of persons as a percentage of 39f; Korean value of unpaid care work and care of persons as a percentage of 39, 39f, 136t, 137; Nicaraguan value of unpaid care work and care of persons as a percentage of 39f; Nicaraguan value of unpaid care work and care of persons compared to 192, 192t; SNA rules for calculating 4; South African value of unpaid care work and care of persons as a percentage of 39, 39f, 40, 89; Tanzanian value of unpaid care work and care of persons as a percentage of 39, 39f, 66; value of unpaid care work and care of persons as a percentage of 39f

H

HIV/AIDS epidemic: calculating care burden in Tanzania 32, 33, 58, 59, 60t, 68; in South Africa 32, 91

household composition/type: in Buenos Aires time spent on care of persons by sex and 213–14, 214t; in Buenos Aires time spent on paid and unpaid work by sex and 2 09, 204–5, 205t, 214; in India time spent on childcare by sex and 108t, 109; in Japan changes in relative share of 2-generation and 3-generation households 155, 156f, 168; in Japan fathers' time use distribution by 155–6, 157f, 158, 163; in Japan mothers' time use distribution by 156, 158t, 162–3; in Japan mothers' time use distribution by employment status and 157, 158–9, 160–1t, 162–3; in Korea time spent on paid and unpaid work by sex and 131, 133t; in Tanzania time spent on paid and unpaid work by sex and 56–7, 56t; and Tobit estimations in respect of care of persons 148, 149t; and Tobit estimations in respect of childcare 150, 150t, 151, 168–9; and Tobit estimations in respect of unpaid care work 114t, 115, 115t, 116, 147t, 148

household expenditure: in India time spent on childcare by sex and 109–10, 110t; in India time spent on SNA and extended SNA by location, sex and 101, 102t; and Tobit estimations in respect of unpaid care work 114t, 115, 115t, 116

household income: Buenos Aires care of persons and household absolute poverty 214, 215t; Buenos Aires paid and unpaid work and household absolute poverty 206–7, 207t, 210; influence on amount of unpaid work 25; in Japan time spent on paid and unpaid work by sex and 146, 146t, 152; in Nicaragua time spent on SNA, paid work and unpaid care work by sex and 185–6, 187t, 194; in South Africa time spent on paid and unpaid work by sex and 79–80, 80t, 84; in Tanzania time spent on paid and unpaid work by sex and 55t, 56; and Tobit estimations in respect of care of persons 27, 28t, 61, 62t, 84, 85t, 148, 149t, 188, 190t; and Tobit estimations in respect of unpaid care work 25, 26t, 62, 63t, 85t, 86, 147t, 148, 188, 189t; *see also* personal income

household position 198–9; care of persons in Buenos Aires by sex and 213, 213t; paid and unpaid care work in Buenos Aires by sex and 204, 204t, 208–9

Human Development Report 2007–2008 11, 15, 22

Hungary 153t, 154

I

ICATUS (International Classification of Activities for Time Use Surveys) 4–5

income: *see* household income; personal income

income tax, value of unpaid work compared to: in Buenos Aires 41f; comparisons between survey countries 40–2, 42f; in India 41, 41f, 42; in Japan 41, 41f; in Korea 41, 41f, 137–8; in Nicaragua 41, 41f, 193; in South Africa 41, 41f, 42, 89; in Tanzania 41, 41f, 66–7

India 92–117; care dependency ratio 33f, 34f; care of sick, elderly and disabled adults 106–7, 106t; caste 97, 100, 108t, 115, 116; classification groups 93–4; comparison of composition of hours spent on SNA and unpaid care work by country and sex 18, 19, 19f; comparison of mean time spent per day by on activities by sub-category of unpaid care work, country and sex 21, 22, 22f; comparison of mean time spent per day on activities by SNA category, country and sex 14–15, 15–16, 15f; comparison of mean time spent per day on activities by SNA category, country and sex for actors 17f; comparison of mean time spent per day on sub-categories of unpaid care work by country and sex for actors 23, 23f; comparison of participation rates by SNA category, country and sex 13, 13f, 14; comparison of participation rates by sub-category of unpaid care work, country and sex 21f; distribution of population by sex and time spent on person care 111–12, 112t; female economic activity rate and share 11t; key determinants of time spent on unpaid care work 114–16; methodology and objectives 8t, 92–4; religion in 97, 100, 109, 116; simultaneous time capture 6, 7; size of survey 92; time allocation across unpaid care work and SNA 94–6, 95t; time recording 5, 7, 93; Tobit estimations on care of persons 27, 28t, 115, 115t; Tobit estimations on unpaid care work 25, 26t, 114–15, 114t; unpaid care work components 105–6, 105t; value of unpaid care work 37, 39, 39f, 40, 41, 41f, 42; *see also* India and time spent on childcare; India socio-economic variables and time distribution across extended SNA and SNA

India and time spent on childcare 107–12; comparison across religious categories 109; mean daily hours spent and participation in childcare-related community services and help to other households 113–14, 113t; mean daily hours spent on subcategories of direct childcare by sex and location 111, 111t; mean hours spent on direct child care by sex and location 107, 107t; time spent and participation by

228 *Index*

demographic and social variables 107–9, 108t; time spent and participation by education and economic variables 109–11, 110t; time spent and participation on household maintenance by presence of children in different age categories 112–13, 113t

India socio-economic variables and time distribution across extended SNA and SNA 96–105; across activity classification groups by sex and location 103–4, 103t; by age, sex and location 29, 97–8, 97t; caste influence on 97, 100; by children in household, sex and location 29–30, 99–100, 99t; distribution of time spent on unpaid care work by sex 104–5, 104f; by educational status, sex and location 100, 101t; by household expenditure, sex and location 101, 102t; by marital status, sex and location 98–9, 98f; religion's influence on 97, 100, 116; by work status and location 31, 102–3, 102t

International Classification of Activities for Time Use Surveys (ICATUS) 4–5

Ireland 22

Ironmonger, D. 6, 20

Italy 16, 43

J

Japan 142–70; care dependency ratio 32, 33, 33f, 34f; comparison of composition of hours spent on SNA and unpaid care work by country and sex 18, 19f; comparison of mean time spent per day by on activities by sub-category of unpaid care work, country and sex 22f; comparison of mean time spent per day on activities by SNA category, country and sex 15f, 16; comparison of mean time spent per day on activities by SNA category, country and sex for actors 17f; comparison of mean time spent per day on sub-categories of unpaid care work by country and sex for actors 23f; comparison of participation rates by SNA category, country and sex 13f, 14; comparison of participation rates by sub-category of unpaid care work, country and sex 20, 21f; methodology for survey 7, 8t, 142–3; sample size 142; simultaneous time capture 6; time recording 5, 6; Tobit estimation on childcare 150, 150t, 168–9; Tobit estimations on care of persons 27, 28t, 148, 149t, 168; Tobit estimations on unpaid care work 25, 26t, 146, 147t, 148, 168; value of unpaid care work 39f, 41, 41f; *see also* Japan and time spent on care for elderly; Japan and time spent on childcare; Japan and time spent on paid and unpaid work

Japan and time spent on care for elderly 163–7; care policies influence on 166–7; caring assistance use influence on 165–6; daily time distribution of men and women providing care for a family member 165, 165t, 169; daily time use distribution of men and women providing care according to use of caring assistance 166, 167t, 169; Long Term Care Insurance (LTCI) 163, 166, 167; percentage of caregivers for family members using care assistance 165, 166f; percentage of men and women who usually care for a family member 163, 164f; percentage of people caring for family members living in separate residence 164f, 165

Japan and time spent on childcare 152–63; changes in relative share of 2-generation and 3-generation households 155, 156f, 168; comparison of daily time use with 12 countries 152, 153t, 154, 168; fathers' time use distribution by household type 155–6, 157f, 158, 163; labour force participation of mothers by household type 156, 159f; labour force participation rate changes for single mothers 159, 161f; mothers' time use distribution by household type 156, 158t, 162–3; mothers' time use distribution by household type and employment status 157, 158–9, 160–1t, 162–3; single mothers' time use data by type of employment 159, 161, 162t, 163; Tobit estimation on 148, 150, 150t, 168–9; trends in daily time use for mothers and fathers 154, 155t; trends in relation to childcare policy 161–3

Japan and time spent on paid and unpaid work 143–52; by age group and sex 144, 144t, 151; distribution of activities over day by sex 143–4, 143t; by household income and sex 146, 146t, 152; by marital status and sex 145, 145t, 151; by presence of children and sex 30, 144, 145t, 146, 151, 152; by work status and sex 145t, 146, 151

K

key concepts 3, 4–7; classifications for unpaid care work 4–5; simultaneous time capture 6–7; time recording methods 5–6

Korean Labour and Income Panel Survey (KLIP) 135, 136

L

labour force surveys 2

Long Term Care Insurance (LTCI) 163, 166, 167

longitudinal data 44

M

Marchand, T. 12

marital status: in India time spent on childcare by sex and 108–9, 108t; in India time spent on SNA and extended SNA by location, sex and 98–9, 98f; in Japan time spent on paid and unpaid work by sex and 145, 145t, 151; in Korea time spent on paid and unpaid work by sex and 129, 130t, 140; in Nicaragua time spent on SNA, paid work and unpaid care work by sex and 183–4, 184t, 194; in South Africa time spent on paid and unpaid work by sex and 76, 76t, 84; in Tanzania time spent on paid and unpaid work by sex and 52, 53t, 54, 59; and Tobit estimations in respect of care of persons 27, 28t, 61, 62t, 84, 85t, 115t, 116, 123, 123t, 124t, 125, 148, 149t, 188, 190t; and Tobit estimations in respect of unpaid care work 25, 26t, 62, 63t, 85t, 86, 114t, 115, 123, 123t, 124t, 125, 147t, 148, 188, 189t

mean actor time 9

mean population time 9

Meena, R. 13

methodology 3, 7–9, 43; in Buenos Aires 7, 8–9, 8t, 197–8; in India 8t, 92–4; in Japan 7, 8t, 142–3; in Korea 7, 8t, 119; in Nicaragua 8t, 173–4; in South Africa 8–9, 8t, 69, 72; summary 8t; in Tanzania 7–8, 8t

N

National Bureau of Statistics (Tanzania) 46

National Standard of Living Survey 1998 (Nicaragua) 172

National Statistics Office (NSO) (Korea) 118, 120, 121, 122, 132, 135, 137, 138

Netherlands 15, 18

Nicaragua 171–96; care dependency ratio 32, 33, 33f, 34f, 186, 187t; care of persons and possible reasons for small time spent on 195; comparison of composition of hours spent on SNA and unpaid care work by country and sex 18, 19, 19f; comparison of mean time spent per day by on activities by sub-category of unpaid care work, country and sex 22f; comparison of mean time spent per day on activities by SNA category, country and sex 15f; comparison of mean time spent per day on activities by SNA category, country and sex for actors 17f; comparison of mean time spent per day on sub-categories of unpaid care work by country and sex for actors 23f; comparison of participation

230 *Index*

rates by SNA category, country and sex 13, 13f, 14; comparison of participation rates by sub-category of unpaid care work, country and sex 21f; defining care work and work 172–3; distribution of time spent on care of persons by sex 180–1, 181f; distribution of time spent on unpaid care work by sex 180, 180f, 194; and domestic workers 186; female economic activity rate and share 11, 11t; fertility rates 33; fuel and water collection 13, 179t; *Human Development Report 2007–8* on childcare 22; methodology for survey 8t, 173–4; simultaneous time capture 6; size of sample 172; survey population description 173–6; time recording 5, 6, 172; Tobit estimations for unpaid care work 26t, 27, 188, 189t, 194–5; Tobit estimations on care of persons 27, 28t, 188, 190t, 191, 194–5; value of unpaid care work and care of persons 37, 38, 191–3, 192t, 195; value of unpaid care work and care of persons as a percentage of GDP 39f; value of unpaid care work and care of persons compared to GDP 1998 192, 192t; value of unpaid care work as a percentage of paid work in economy 40, 41f, 193; value of unpaid care work compared to income tax 41, 41f, 193; *see also* Nicaragua work-care regimes participation rate and mean time spent on selected activities

Nicaragua work-care regimes participation rate and mean time spent on selected activities: by activity and sex 185, 186t, 195; by age group and sex 29, 182–3, 183t, 194; by conjugal status and sex 183–4, 184t, 194; by location and sex 181–2, 182t, 194; by monetary household income quintile and sex 185–6, 187t, 194; by number of children under 6 and sex 30, 184–5, 185t, 194; participation rates, mean actor time and mean population time by SNA category and sex 177–8, 178t, 194; participation rates, mean actor time and mean population time in SNA work by sex 178, 179t; participation rates, mean participant time and mean population time in unpaid care work by sex 178, 179t, 180; time use distribution indicators 177

Norway 15, 153t

P

Pacholok, S. 15, 25, 43
participation rate 9
personal income 27; in Korea 121; in South Africa 71, 79, 79t, 83, 84; *see also* household income
Philippines 18
Picchio, A. 171
policy xxi, 1, 42; influence in Japan on care of elderly 166–7; influence in Japan on childcare 161–3
Political and Social Economy of Care 2, 4
poverty: in Buenos Aires 199–200; in Buenos Aires time spent on care of persons by sex and household absolute 214, 215t; in Buenos Aires time spent on paid and unpaid work by sex and household absolute 206–7, 207t, 210

R

race factors: and Tobit estimations in respect of care of persons 27, 28t, 84, 85t; and Tobit estimations in respect of unpaid care work 25, 26t, 85t, 86
religion in India 97, 100, 109, 116
Republic of Korea 118–41; care dependency ratio 32, 33, 33f, 34f, 121; comparison of composition of hours spent on SNA and unpaid care work by country and sex 18, 19f; comparison of mean time spent per day by on activities by sub-category of unpaid care work, country and sex 22f; comparison of mean time spent per day on activities by SNA category, country and sex 15f, 16; comparison of mean time spent per day on activities

by SNA category, country and sex for actors 17f; comparison of mean time spent per day on sub-categories of unpaid care work by country and sex for actors 23f; comparison of participation rates by SNA category, country and sex 13f, 14; comparison of participation rates by sub-category of unpaid care work, country and sex 21f; defining paid and unpaid work 121–2; distribution of time spent on person care 132–3, 134f, 135f; distribution of time spent on unpaid care work 131–2, 133, 134f, 135f; female economic activity rate and share 11t; key deteriminants of time spent on care 122–5; Korean Labour and Income Panel Survey (KLIP) 135, 136; methodology for survey 7, 8t, 119; size of sample 118–19; survey descriptions 1999 and 2004 119–21; time recording 5, 6, 7, 119; time spent on activities by sex in 1999 and 2004 122t; Tobit estimations on care of persons 27, 28t, 122–5, 123t, 124t; Tobit estimations on unpaid care work 25, 26t, 122–4, 123t, 124t; total hours spent on unpaid care work, person care and paid work 138–9, 139t; value of unpaid care work and person care 37, 133–9, 140–1; value of unpaid care work and person care as percentage of GDP 39, 39f, 136t, 137; value of unpaid care work and person care by year 137, 137t; value of unpaid care work compared to income tax 41, 41f, 137–8; *see also* Republic of Korea time spent on paid work and unpaid care work

Republic of Korea time spent on paid work and unpaid care work 125–31; by age group and sex 29, 126–7, 127t, 139; by children in household and sex 30, 129–30, 131t, 140; by education and sex 1999 and 2004 127–9, 128t, 139–40; by household composition and sex 131, 133t; by marital status and sex 129, 130t, 140; by sex 1999 and 2004 125–6, 125t, 139, 140; by work status and sex 31, 130–1, 132t, 140

S
settlement type: in India mean hours spent by actors on SNA and extended SNA by sex and location 95–6, 96f; in Nicaragua time spent on SNA, paid work and unpaid care work by sex and 181–2, 182t, 194; in South Africa time spent on paid and unpaid work by sex and 78–9, 78t, 83, 84; in Tanzania time spent on paid and unpaid work by sex and 55t, 56; and Tobit estimations in respect of care of persons 27, 28, 28t, 61, 62t, 188, 190t; and Tobit estimations in respect of unpaid care work 26t, 62, 63t, 114t, 115, 115t, 116, 188, 189t; *see also* India socio-economic variables and time distribution across extended SNA and SNA
sick, care of: and care of elderly and disabled in India 106–7, 106t; in Tanzania 58, 59, 60t
simultaneous time capture 6–7
single mothers: labour force participation rate changes for single mothers 159, 161f; time use data by type of employment in Japan 159, 161, 162t, 163; and Tobit estimations in respect of childcare 150, 150t
Slovenia 153t
Smeeding, M. 12, 168
SNA (System of National Accounts) 4; SNA-related categories 12–19
social reproduction 171
South Africa 69–91; care dependency ratio 33f, 34f; care of persons and paid work 80–3, 81t; care of persons in detail 83–4; comparison of composition of hours spent on SNA and unpaid care work by country and sex 18, 19, 19f; comparison of mean time spent per day on activities by SNA category, country and sex

14, 15f; comparison of mean time spent per day on activities by SNA category, country and sex for actors 17f; comparison of mean time spent per day on activities by sub-category of unpaid care work, country and sex 21–2, 22f; comparison of mean time spent per day on sub-categories of unpaid care work by country and sex for actors 23f; comparison of participation rates by SNA category, country and sex 13–14, 13f; comparison of participation rates by sub-category of unpaid care work, country and sex 20, 21f; distribution of time spent on person care 87, 87t; distribution of time spent on unpaid care work by sex 86–7, 86t; female economic activity rate and share 11t; fuel and water collection 72; HIV/AIDS epidemic 32, 91; key determinants of time spent on care 84–5; macro measures to calculate size of care economy 89–90; methodology for survey 8–9, 8t, 69, 72; population 69; simultaneous time capture 6, 7; standard dependency ratio 32; survey population description 69–71; Tobit estimations on care of persons 27, 28t, 84–5, 85t; Tobit estimations on unpaid care work 25, 26t, 85t, 86; value for unpaid care work and person care 38, 87–9, 88t; value of unpaid care work and care of persons as a percentage of GDP 39, 39f, 40, 89; value of unpaid care work compared to income tax 41, 41f, 42, 89; value of unpaid care work compared to value of government social services 89–90; *see also* South Africa time spent on paid and unpaid work

South Africa time spent on paid and unpaid work 72–80; by age group and sex 29, 75–6, 75t; by children in household and sex 30, 76–7, 77t, 84; distribution of activities over day by sex 72–3, 73t; and domestic workers 78, 79; by household income and sex 79–80, 80t, 84; by marital status and sex 76, 76t, 84; by personal income and sex 79, 79t, 83, 84; by population group and sex 74–5, 75t; by settlement type and sex 78–9, 78t, 83, 84; by sex 73–4, 74t, 80–1; by work status and sex 31, 77t, 78, 84

standard dependency ratio 31–2
Statistics South Africa 69
stylised approach to time recording 5
Survey on Time Use and Leisure Activities (STULA) (Japan) 142, 143, 155, 156, 159, 163
Sweden 15, 16, 43, 153t
System of National Accounts (SNA): *see* SNA (System of National Accounts)

T

Tanzania 46–68; care dependency ratio 33, 33f, 34, 34f; care of persons and paid work 57–8, 58f; care of persons in detail 58–61, 60t; care of sick 58, 59, 60t; comparison of composition of hours spent on SNA and unpaid care work by country and sex 18, 19f; comparison of mean time spent per day on activities by SNA category, country and sex 15, 15f, 16; comparison of mean time spent per day on activities by SNA category, country and sex for actors 17f; comparison of mean time spent per day on activities by sub-category of unpaid care work, country and sex 21, 22f, 23; comparison of mean time spent per day on sub-categories of unpaid care work by country and sex for actors 23, 23f; comparison of participation rates by SNA category, country and sex 12–13, 13f, 14; comparison of participation rates by sub-category of unpaid care work, country and sex 20, 21f; data from Integrated Labour Force Survey (ILFS) 46; distribution of time spent on activities per day by sex 46–7,

Index 233

47t; distribution of time spent on person care by sex 64f, 65; distribution of time spent on unpaid work by sex 64, 64f; female economic activity rate and share 11t; fertility rates 33; fuel and water collection 48–9; HIV/AIDS epidemic 32, 33, 58, 59, 60t, 68; key determinants of time spent on care 61–3, 62t, 63t; methodology 7–8, 8t; population 46; simultaneous time capture 6, 7; size of sample 46; standard dependency ratio 32; survey population description 47–50; time recording 5, 6, 7; Tobit estimations on care of persons 27, 28t, 61, 62t; Tobit estimations on unpaid care work 25, 26t, 62–3, 63t; value of unpaid care work 37–8, 65–7; value of unpaid care work and care of persons as a percentage of GDP 39, 39f, 66; value of unpaid care work compared to income tax 41, 41f, 66–7; *see also* Tanzania time spent on paid and unpaid work

Tanzania time spent on paid and unpaid work 50–7; by age group and sex 29, 52, 52t, 59; by co-residence with young children and sex 53t, 54, 59; domestic worker classification 54; by educational achievement status and sex 55t, 56, 61; by household composition and sex 56–7, 56t; by household income and sex 55t, 56; by marital status and sex 52, 53t, 54, 59; percentage of people doing person care and paid work by sex 57–8, 58f; by settlement type and sex 55t, 56; time spent by sex 51–2, 51f; by work status and sex 31, 53t, 54

time recording: diary approach 5–6; mean actor time measure 9; mean population time measure 9; simultaneous time capture 6–7; stylised approach 5

Tobit estimations 3, 24–7; care of persons summary of results 25, 27, 28t; India care of persons 27, 28t, 115, 115t; India unpaid care work 25, 26t, 114–15, 114t; Japan care of persons 27, 28t, 148, 149t, 168; Japan childcare 148, 150, 150t, 168–9; Japan unpaid care work 25, 26t, 146, 147t, 148, 168; Korea care of persons 27, 28t, 122–5, 123t, 124t; Korea unpaid care work 25, 26t, 122–4, 123t, 124t; Nicaragua care of persons 27, 28t, 188, 190t, 191, 194–5; Nicaragua unpaid care work 26t, 27, 188, 189t, 194–5; South Africa care of persons 27, 28t, 84–5, 85t, 90; South Africa unpaid care work 25, 26t, 85t, 86, 90; Tanzania care of persons 27, 28t, 61, 62t; Tanzania unpaid care work 25, 26t, 62–3, 63t; unpaid care work summary of results 24–5, 26t

U

United Kingdom 153t
United Nations Development Programme (UNDP) 15, 16, 18, 22, 33, 35
United States of America 10, 11, 153t

V

value of unpaid care work and person care 34–42; approaches to measuring hourly earnings 35–8; as compared to government expenditure on social services 67, 89–90, 138, 141, 193; comparisons with macroeconomic indicators 38–42; as a percentage of paid work in economy 40–1, 41f, 193; *see also* Gross Domestic Product; income tax, value of unpaid work compared to

W

Wage Structure Survey of Ministry of Labour 134–6
Wajcman, J. 5, 16
Wolf, D. 36, 41
work status: in Buenos Aires time spent on care of persons by sex and 211, 212t, 213; in Buenos Aires time spent on paid and unpaid work by sex and 29, 203–4,

203t, 208; gender combined with 30–1; in India time spent on childcare by sex and 110–11, 110t; in India time spent on SNA and unpaid care work by location, sex and 31, 102–3, 102t; in Japan mothers' time use distribution by household type and 157, 158–9, 160–1t, 162–3; in Japan time spent on paid and unpaid work by sex and 145t, 146, 151; in Korea time spent on paid and unpaid work by sex and 31, 130–1, 132t, 140; in South Africa time spent on paid and unpaid work by sex and 31, 77t, 78, 84; in Tanzania time spent on paid and unpaid work by sex and 53t, 54, 59; and Tobit estimations in respect of care of persons 61, 62t, 85, 85t, 123, 123t; and Tobit estimations in respect of childcare 150t, 151; and Tobit estimations in respect of unpaid care work 25, 26t, 62, 63t, 85t, 86, 114t, 115, 123, 123t, 124t

World's Women 1995: Trends and Statistics 10

For Product Safety Concerns and Information please contact our EU representative GPSR@taylorandfrancis.com
Taylor & Francis Verlag GmbH, Kaufingerstraße 24, 80331 München, Germany

www.ingramcontent.com/pod-product-compliance
Lightning Source LLC
Chambersburg PA
CBHW050439240426
43661CB00055B/2443